See Jane Climb

HOW COMPETITIVE STAIR CLIMBING CHANGED MY LIFE

Jane Trahanovsky

Harish –
To a sweet and gentle soul. I'm so proud to call you step-brother. Thank you being part of my story. I hope to climb with you again soon.
xo Jane
5·30·16

Published by
Duswalt Press
280 N. Westlake Blvd Suite 110
Westlake Village, CA 91362
www.duswaltpress.com

Manufactured in the United States of America, or in the United Kingdom when distributed elsewhere.

Trahanovsky, Jane
    See Jane Climb
How Competitive Stair Climbing Changed My Life

    ISBN:
    Paperback: 978–1938015–37–3
    eBook: 978–1938015–38–0

Cover design by: Jeff Barton
Cover photo by: Josh Telles
Interior design: Scribe Inc

This book is dedicated to you
if you think you can't.

You can.

"The thief comes to steal and destroy. I came that they may have and enjoy life, and have it in abundance [to the full, till it overflows]."

John 10:10, Amplified Bible

ACKNOWLEDGMENTS

Thank you to my brother Mark Trahanovsky for introducing me to the wacky and wonderful world of competitive stair climbing. It was you who suggested that I write a book about stair climbing in early 2011, after I had written an article for a local paper. You always plant seeds that bring growth in my life.

Thank you to my beautiful daughter, Ariana Longley. When you decided to move to Scotland in September of 2011 to pursue your master's degree, you gave me the courage to begin this journey. The bravery you displayed in starting life anew in a foreign country inspired me to do something big in my life. You are also my main motivation for staying fit and healthy and wanting to hang around planet Earth for a good long while.

Thank you, Tera McFarland, my friend since the first grade, for your encouragement during the early stages of the project. I asked you to read through what I had written to see if it was worth reading, and you kept me moving forward with your support.

To Hollye Dexter, thank you for your honest criticism of my first fifty pages. Your editing was invaluable and helped make the finished product what it is.

To my editor and sister in Christ, Claudia Volkman, thank you for your gentle spirit and enormous patience throughout the editing process. You are a gift.

Thank you, Karen Strauss, my publisher, for your confidence in the book and for your knowledge and wisdom in answering the many questions this "newbie" threw out. Thank you for connecting me with Claudia. She is a perfect fit.

Special thanks to Craig Batley, Art Streiber, Josh Telles, Norman Schwartz, Jason Hughes, and Jeff Barton. The book would not be the same without any of you.

Finally, my unending gratitude goes to my enormous "stepfamily," the global stair-climbing community. Each of you who make it to the top is a treasure, inspiring those around you with your strength and a story uniquely yours. You are irreplaceable. Stair climbing would not be the same without you. Keep on climbing!

CONTENTS

FOREWORD FROM HAROLD P. WIMMER

National President and CEO, American Lung Association

There are many reasons that someone chooses to become involved in a stair climb. For many, the idea of climbing five floors of stairs, much less upwards of one hundred floors, is daunting, both physically and mentally. And to take this on, most are motivated by a mission. Jane Trahanovsky, whose journey took her from a non-climber to one of the top fifty female climbers in the U.S. for the past two seasons, shares her motivation and passion for stair climbing throughout the chapters of this inspiring and entertaining book.

As National President and CEO of the American Lung Association, I know that tens of thousands of our constituents climb for other reasons. We hold more than fifty Fight For Air Climbs in some of the tallest buildings nationwide every year. With more than 33 million Americans suffering from lung disease, most of them are motivated by a desire to help in the fight against asthma, COPD, and lung cancer. They're climbing and raising funds to help family, friends, and loved ones who struggle to breathe. In fact, in the past two years alone, Fight For Air Climbers have raised nearly $20,000,000 for lung disease research and education. Many of them are also motivated by a desire to challenge themselves athletically. Jane was one of those climbers at our Las Vegas Climb event.

Jane does a nice job of describing the camaraderie, fun, physical challenge, and energy of stair climbs. This unique event gives every climber a sense of the lung power needed to climb and what it feels like when one is literally fighting for air—which is what someone with lung disease experiences every day.

Jane's honesty about her own physical and psychological hurdles to becoming part of the "step-family" is inspiring. I think many of us can relate our own fitness challenges to much of what she shares. Sometimes the hardest part of the climb is just getting to the building and lacing up the shoes. Jane gives us a great example of pushing through her fear and anxiety and taking that first step toward what has become a lifelong passion for her.

As you read these pages, I would encourage everyone to follow Jane's lead and participate in an American Lung Association Fight For Air Climb in your area. You can find one at www.FightForAirClimb.org. We invite you to experience the thrill of stepping up to this challenge and, at the same time, raising funds for much-needed research that helps everyone breathe easier.

As Jane knows, whether you're a first-time climber or a stair-climb veteran—to climb successfully it's important to train before the big event. Stair climbing is a great sport that improves your fitness and burns more calories than walking or running. And as always, be sure to consult your doctor before beginning any new fitness routine.

Consider these expert tips as you get started:

- Start slow. If you are new to climbing stairs, then start slow and build up your pace.
- To reduce the risk of injury, place your entire foot on the stair each time.
- Experiment with climbing techniques. For example, some climbers prefer to keep their arms by their sides, while others prefer to use the handrails. You can climb one or two steps at a time, depending on your comfort level. Use your training climbs to find what works for you.
- Carrying water with you can impede your climbing. Keep in mind that on event day, there are normally water stops and water available at the finish line.
- Consider a light snack a few minutes before the climb begins. This will help you maintain your energy level without feeling sick.
- Cool down. When you reach the top, take a couple of minutes to cool down and stretch. This will help keep your muscles from being too sore.

I congratulate Jane and everyone who climbs competitively, for a charitable cause, for better fitness, or just for fun. Hopefully this book will inspire you to take your first climb. It's an experience you must not miss!

I don't remember most of the conversation, but I do recall my younger brother Mark calling me in November 2007 to tell me about his latest stair climbing conquest, the Sears Tower (now Willis Tower) in Chicago. At some point during the call, he suggested that I should participate in an upcoming stair climb at the AON building in Los Angeles the following April. I remember replying, "Why would I want to do that?" He said he was helping recruit climbers since it was a brand-new climb that would raise money for a charity. I said I'd think about it.

Mark made sure that I did the climb. There was no way I could ever have imagined how big a step I was taking when I set foot in the stairwell that day. It was the first of 1,393 steps I took to the top of a sixty-two-story building, and those steps changed my life forever. I was fifty-one years old, five feet four-and-three-quarters inches tall, and weighed well over 220 pounds at the time. In the two years following, I lost eighty pounds without ever setting foot in a gym, without eating special "diet" foods or spending money on supplements, without investing in anything other than my time and a good pair of running shoes. In doing so, I found true freedom. I changed my life by eating less and exercising more— I lost fifty pounds in eight months, and over eighty pounds in two years. By following the same basic eating plan and staying active, I continue to maintain a healthy weight.

According to current statistics from the Centers for Disease Control (CDC), 69 percent of America's adult population is overweight; 35 percent of that population is obese. More than 18 percent of children ages six to nineteen are overweight. The United States has the second most overweight population in the world among large countries. We were the fattest but were overtaken by Mexico a couple of years ago. (We didn't get slimmer; they got heavier). The World Health Organization (WHO) states that in 2014 more than 600 million of the world's adults were obese and nearly two billion were overweight. Forty-two million children younger than five were overweight or obese in 2013. *Forty-two million* overweight young children! The world's overweight population has doubled since 1980. Too many people are sedentary and eat convenience foods that taste good because they are full of fat, sugar, and salt.

Stair climbing has become my passion and motivation for staying fit, so one purpose in writing this book is to introduce the little-known but fast-growing sport of competitive stair climbing. More important, though, is my desire to promote physical activity—and perhaps even stair climbing—as part of an overall fitness program. I've also included the stories of some of the wonderful athletes who make up the competitive stair climbing community across the country and around the world. I am humbled to be a member of this family of unique individuals who are so completely devoted to remaining active, healthy, and youthful.

The global stair climbing community is a group as diverse as the general population itself. They are the nicest athletes on the planet; most of them are "everyday athletes"—average people with a passion for an unusual sport. I have been moved to tears by many of their stories. My "step"-siblings (as we refer to each other) are students, retirees, engineers, lawyers, teachers, and single parents, as well as personal trainers and fitness buffs. We have a doorman from New York City on our team, a male flight attendant, and a fatal crash analyst for the California Highway Patrol. One climber works for Groupon; another teaches blind teenagers. At least two climbers I know don't own a car. Our common passion for pushing our minds and bodies beyond ordinary limits has transformed thousands of climbers into an intimate "stepfamily," with a little help from social media.

I sincerely hope that through our stories you will be inspired to adopt an active lifestyle and overcome any challenges holding you back from being fit, healthy, and happy.

I explore my childhood and past experiences in the pages ahead not to place blame or with any motivation other than to explain how my upbringing shaped me. We are all products of genetics and environment. Each member of my family has a different perspective on events that took place over the years. I would not be the person I am today, for better or for worse, if I hadn't experienced all that I have in my lifetime.

It's one thing to read about getting fit, but it's quite another to put a plan into action, do the work, and make the sacrifices needed to bring about change. If you eat like the average person, you'll be an average person. Many people have told me that I'm an inspiration, but few of them have done anything to bring about change in their own lives. My one regret is that I didn't make these changes earlier in my life. Please don't wait another minute to start on your own personal journey to getting fit. If I did it, you can, too.

First Steps

I never actually agreed to participate in my first stair climb. My younger brother Mark started competitive stair climbing in September of 2007 at the age of forty-nine. He phoned me in November 2007 after completing a climb at Chicago's Sears Tower (now the Willis Tower). The Sears Tower is the country's tallest building, and this was Mark's second competitive climb.

I'm caught off-guard when he asks during the call if I want to do the upcoming April AON climb in Los Angeles. Mark has been a runner for years, has done numerous 5Ks, and is trim and athletic. I am not. I'm fifty-one years old and, at five feet four and three-quarter inches, weigh in at well over 220 pounds. I don't know how much I really weigh. I won't get on the scale—it's too depressing. The last time I was weighed at the doctor's office, I stepped on the scale backward so I wouldn't have to see the numbers. I learned that trick from an overweight friend. That, dear reader, is what's known as *denial.*

I respond to Mark's invitation with sarcasm: "Why would I want to do that?" He says it's a new climb and he's helping to recruit climbers. He adds that funds raised by the climb will go to charity. I tell him I'll think about it. I hang up and think, *The last thing I'd ever dream of doing would be climbing a tall building. Mark is crazy.* I don't give our conversation another thought.

One night a week or so later Mark calls me to say he's on his way to my house with his old treadmill. He says I can use it to train for the climb; he assures me that I don't necessarily have to train on stairs to be a good stair climber. Apparently Mark thinks I'm doing the AON climb. I take the treadmill. I'll use it; I know I don't get enough physical activity. Thankfully, my nineteen year-old daughter, Ariana, is away at college—because the only place the treadmill will fit is in her room. When she comes home to visit, she'll have to walk over it to reach her bed. Great.

I start running on the treadmill for about thirty minutes several days a week. I'm a single mom, and Ariana is my only child, so I can pound away on the treadmill early in the morning before I go to work and not bother anyone. I watch the KTLA morning show on Ariana's little TV while I run, and the time passes fairly quickly.

When I finally do sign up online for the climb some months later, after repeated calls from Mark asking if I've signed up yet, I send out an email to the eighteen people in our office, inviting them to join me. It would be fun, not to mention less scary, to go as a team. Several coworkers say they're up for the challenge, but as the day draws near, I have no teammates. A few days before the event, my boss Craig asks who's going with me, and I tell him no one. Craig is eight years older than I am, in great shape, works out with a trainer, and is a devout juicer. He has never done a stair climb either. He feels sorry for me going alone, so he says he'll do the climb. He figures if I can do it, he can do it. I am happy to have company.

Just before 8:00 a.m. on April 26, 2008, Craig and I approach downtown Los Angeles on our way to the climb. He lives nearby and offers to drive. I'm glad because I'm so stressed I don't think I can make the hour-long trek from Orange County by myself. Just driving into LA is daunting as the city skyline comes into view. There it is: the big, black, foreboding AON building looming on the horizon. At sixty-two stories, it's the second tallest building in Los Angeles, and we will climb sixty-three stories to finish on the roof. The AON building was the tallest structure in Los Angeles (and in the state of California) until 1989 when the U.S. Bank Tower was completed. The large red AON logo displayed atop the building honors the skyscraper's anchor tenant, the AON Corporation.

Today when I see the building against the mountains in the background, little pains shoot up the insides of my arms like electrical shocks. Maybe I'll have a heart attack and won't have to climb. How did I end up here? What was I thinking? There's no way I can do this. I'm petrified. I'm so worried about the climb that I slept only a few hours the night before. I'm wearing my glasses because my eyes are so irritated from lack of sleep that I can't wear contacts. I *hate* wearing glasses.

I've been praying that I'll finish—and that I won't be the last one to the top. I figure I can make it eventually, but I don't have a clue how long it will take, and I'm afraid I'll be last. My brother says he thinks there's a woman climbing who has only one leg and jokes that I should at least be able to beat her. Funny guy, my brother. Mark likes to call stair climbing "the hardest sport you've never heard of."

Craig and I arrive at the climb registration center and sign the necessary forms. Climbers must sign waivers in order to compete, agreeing to hold the building owners and/or management harmless in case of injury, and we also complete a form with emergency contact information.

As competitive as the sport has become, most climbs in the United States are promoted not as races but as fund-raising events. Proceeds from today's entry fees and fund-raising benefit today's sponsor, the American Lung Association (ALA). The ALA sponsors climbs in sixty-five U.S. cities, more than any other organization.

I find Mark in the crowd. This is his seventh stair climb since September. In February, he did the Denver ALA climb. There, he started out too fast and had a rough time, but he's excited to compete today and introduces me to some of the other climbers. Two of them make a lasting impression on me. Tim Van Orden is video taping interviews for his website, runningraw.com. Tim, who eats nothing but raw food, is the person who introduced Mark to stair climbing. Craig and I agree to appear on Tim's video, and he asks us some questions on camera.

I also meet forty-two-year-old Jeff Dinkin, who is terribly banged up from a cycling accident earlier in the week. He has a sling on one arm and road rash all over his arms and legs, but he is nevertheless exuberant about participating today. Jeff's first climb, like Mark's, was the U.S. Bank Climb in September.

I am assigned bib number 151. What a coincidence! This is my first climb, and I'm fifty-one years old. We're given timing chips to affix to our shoes. The chip registers the time a racer crosses over a mat at the start and again at the finish. The folks at the starting line send climbers off ten to fifteen seconds apart to avoid creating congestion in the stairwells. I'm terrified as we take our place in line for the start. Mark, Tim, Jeff, and other fast climbers line up first to take off. I'm farther back in line, which is fine with me. I'm in no hurry to do this.

I say now that your first climb is the best because you have absolutely no idea what you're in for. The most stairs I had climbed at any one time before was as a freshman at the University of Pittsburgh in 1974. I was meeting with my advisor after classes. His office was about twenty stories up in the beautiful Cathedral of Learning on Pitt's main campus. I arrived to find the elevator broken and a sign directing people to the stairs. I was furious, wondering how they could "make" people climb that far—ridiculous! I recall stopping on a landing part way up to try and catch my breath. I wished I had worn more suitable shoes, not the slippery sandals I had on. By the time I got to my advisor's floor, I was red-faced and huffing and puffing. I had to stand outside until I could breathe normally;

I was too embarrassed to walk in gasping for air. It was awful doing those stairs then—and I was eighteen years old and more than eighty pounds lighter than I am this morning.

Years earlier, I worked at a restaurant in Anaheim, in a three-story turn-of-the-century home. At the time I was accustomed to doing stairs. As a server I would carry heavy trays full of food up a flight of stairs to the second floor, run to the basement for supplies, and make an occasional trip to the office on the third floor. Later on, as a manager, my office was on the third floor, which required multiple trips daily to and from the kitchen and dining room on the first floor to the basement to check on wines, and so on. We used to laugh at salespeople who came up from the first floor to the third floor panting and out of breath. Pity I hadn't worked there since 2003—I'd be better prepared for today.

Climbers enter the stairwell via a doorway on an outside corner of the building. Craig starts before I do, but I'm too nerve-wracked to notice when he went into the stairwell or wonder how he's doing. I get the go-ahead to start, and I take off at a trot. I am really scared. My heart is beating so hard and so rapidly, I think it will burst from my chest, and I haven't climbed one step yet. I can feel my pulse throbbing in my throat. I start up the drab stairwell, taking one step at a time. It's boring—each flight of stairs is the same. My legs feel heavy, and I'm breathing as hard as I have ever breathed in my life. By the time I reach the tenth floor, my mouth is so dry I can barely swallow. Why didn't I drink more water this morning?

Soon after, I pass a couple of women struggling to go on. One is heavyset and leaning against the wall with an anguished look on her face, and the other is trying to console her. At this point, I know I won't be last, so I relax a bit. This is tough, though, and I've barely begun. I still have more than fifty floors to go. The quad muscles above my knees are burning so badly, I want to turn around and run down a few stairs to release the tension. (I later learn that working the muscles harder than usual causes a build-up of lactic acid in the muscle tissue, creating a burning sensation.) The only thing that keeps me from turning around and going back down a few stairs is the knowledge that I'll have even more steps to climb if I do. No matter how hard I breathe, my body still begs for more oxygen. My lungs are burning, and I cannot get enough air.

Gym owner and teammate PJ Glassey put it best in an interview after the 2010 Willis Tower Climb in Chicago:

> Your brain is getting messages from the legs saying there's too much
> acid, plus you're way overheated, then the brain says, "Let's check
> the lungs," and the lungs can't keep up. So the brain checks the heart

which says, "I'm givin' it all I got, Cap'n." Finally brain says "I'm making an executive decision, and it's time to shut it all down."

Seasoned climbers are able to push through this "wall" to finish well. I'm not experienced enough or in good enough shape to be able to do anything like that. I have to step out at the landings to catch my breath quite a few times. I feel very limited by my body; I'm so out of shape. It's a terrible feeling.

There are volunteers stationed every ten floors or so with cups of water, and I pause for a drink a couple of times. At one point I don't think I can go on. Maybe I'll take one of the exits and quit. They have signs on the doors on each floor indicating which floors have actual exits, but by the time I reach one of those floors, I am so near the top that I figure I might just as well stick it out and finish. I'm not willing to admit that I can't do this. I don't want to disappoint Mark or Craig. Or myself.

When I finally see daylight at the end of the stairway ahead, I'm so elated to have made it to the top that I run across the mat at the finish so my timing chip will register and then stop. I go to the railing, but there are people ahead of me yelling, "Come on, hurry up!" and I lumber past the volunteers at the finish. This is one of few climbs in the U.S. that actually ends on the roof. Climbers are allowed to pose for photos on the helipad and soak in sweeping views of the beautiful LA basin.

I look for my brother Mark. He's on the other side of the roof talking to fellow climbers. He looks relieved to see me. He says he was concerned because he waited quite a while for me to emerge from the stairwell. Mark comments that my glasses are fogged up because I'm so overheated. Tell me about it—I'm soaked with sweat. My face is flushed from the exertion.

Craig is on the helipad, which sits about four feet above the surrounding roof area. As soon as I'm able, I climb a few more steps to join him and take in the view. He looks like he just went for a walk in the park; his appearance doesn't give any evidence that this was strenuous for him. I'm speechless, kind of stunned by the whole experience. This is arguably the single hardest thing I've ever done in my life, aside from giving birth to my daughter in 1988—and that was unavoidable and involved a strong painkiller. It takes several minutes for my breathing to return to normal, a bit longer for my heart rate to do so. Surprisingly I'm not sore, but I am completely drained.

Craig also says he's been waiting there for long time. I'm a little miffed. It doesn't seem like it took me *that* long. Craig and I pose for photos and then head back down into the building. Volunteers cut the timing chips from our shoes and tell us to walk down several flights to catch the elevator to the ground floor. I hear Craig say, "Um . . . we've gone too far." We passed the floor with the elevator. Now we have to turn around and go back up another three or four floors. More stairs. I am not at all amused.

Craig's time is 16:15, which is good enough for a second place AG (age group) finish on his very first climb. My time is 34:14. I guess Craig *had* been waiting up there for a while—it took me more than twice as long to finish as it took him. Mark finishes ninth overall with 10:55, garnering a first place finish in his age group. Jeff Dinkin manages to best Mark by seven seconds even though he couldn't use his arms. Tommy Coleman, who won his very first stair climb, the 2006 U.S. Bank Climb, wins the event with a time of 8:17, two seconds faster than Tim, the runningraw.com athlete. Chicago's Jesse Berg, one of the country's top climbers, finishes third with 8:24.

I develop a deep, croupy cough almost immediately after going back down to ground level. Mark tells me that lots of climbers experience this type of cough for at least a few hours after a strenuous climb; sometimes it lasts until the next day. The labored breathing seems to make your lungs open up right down to the tiny capillaries. Some climbers think it loosens up tiny particles of pollutants, such as dust particles, that have been lying dormant, causing your lungs to try to expel them. Some think it's caused by the dust and dirt inhaled while climbing. I think it has more to do with humidity, or a combination of some of the above. It seems the drier the air, the more climbers have the "hack." My throat is dry and sore from breathing so hard.

My first thought when I got to the top at AON was, *I could have done better.* I considered every stop I made, every person I hesitated to pass, how I could have gone faster if I'd trained harder, and so on. I knew at that moment I'd been bitten by the stair-climbing bug, and I was determined to do better on the next climb. Afterward I ask Mark when there will be another climb, and he tells me the next Los Angeles area climb is the U.S. Bank event in late September. I have five months to train.

As difficult as today's climb was, however, my life's journey up until today had been much tougher than climbing any tall building.

CHAPTER TWO

Stepping into the Past

I didn't always have a problem with being overweight. Photos of me up to the age of about nine or ten reveal a skinny, almost anorexic-looking child: knobby-kneed with a "Dutch Boy" haircut. My tumultuous childhood filled me with fear, though, and changed me into a young girl who struggled not only with her weight, but with shame and self-esteem issues as well.

My mom, Sara Jane, was a stay-at-home mom, as were most all mothers in the sixties. There weren't many working moms in our community; those who worked outside the home were typically teachers, nurses, school bus drivers, and bank tellers.

My dad, Nicholas Alexander, was an osteopathic physician and surgeon in the small town of Conemaugh, Pennsylvania, where he was born in 1924, the eldest child of Samuel and Mary (Brumersky) Trahanovsky. My grandfather worked for Bethlehem Steel, like the majority of the male population in Johnstown and the surrounding areas at that time. My dad graduated a year early from high school and went directly to the University of Pittsburgh, where he was enrolled year round and graduated three years later. He wanted to go to medical school, but according to my grandparents' account, many wealthy families sent their sons to medical school to keep them from being drafted during World War II, and as a result there were no spots available for my dad in a traditional medical school. He decided to go instead to the Kansas City School of Osteopathy, where he got his degree in osteopathic medicine.

When I was in fourth grade, a classmate asked how my dad could be a doctor if he wasn't an MD. I said he was a DO. When he asked the difference between and MD and a DO, I told him if he went to an MD and said his back hurt, an MD would give him a pain pill that would make him feel better, but if he told my dad his back hurt, he would give him an osteopathic treatment that would fix his back so it wouldn't hurt anymore. My dad loved my definition. He met my mom during his surgical residency at Lancaster Osteopathic Hospital.

Mom was born in Lancaster, Pennsylvania, to Joseph and Kathryn (Munson) Welk. My grandfather worked as a lineman for Bell of Pennsylvania for fifty years. Mom was born in 1932, the fourth of nine children, seven girls and two boys. My parents met when she was eighteen, my dad twenty-six. According to my mom, who worked at the hospital as a nurse's aide part time her senior year of high school, my dad was known there as "The Mad Russian" due to his terrible temper. He was a perfectionist. There were two ways of doing things—his way and the wrong way. It's been said that to be a successful surgeon one must have a God-complex. It was certainly true of my dad. He was an exceptionally intelligent man with a fantastic sense of humor, the worst temper of anyone I've ever known, and an overly healthy ego. My brothers and I once found a high school textbook of his. Inside the front flap, he'd signed his name as "Nicholas Alexander Sylvester Brumersky Trahanovsky." When we asked him about it, he said the two extra names made his name look more impressive.

My mom and dad met in 1950 and were married a year later. My parents had six children, starting with Kathy in 1952. She was an exceptional child. She could sit up and feed herself before she was four months old. My mom said they didn't like to eat out with her because Kathy attracted so much attention. A man in a restaurant once asked my parents if she was a midget because she was so tiny to be using utensils.

When she was four months old, Kathy got a cold, which turned into pneumonia. She ran a high fever and went into convulsions. My parents rushed her to the hospital in the car, but by the time they got there, she had suffered permanent brain damage. She never developed mentally beyond the age of two, and she spent her entire life in a crib. Kathy required "round the clock" care, which my parents decided they would provide at home. All of her meals were pureed; she wasn't able to chew food. Most often Kathy's meals were jars of baby food, but sometimes she ate regular food, if it was soft and fine textured: mashed potatoes with butter or gravy, warm soup, hot cereal, and so forth.

Once, when I was in my early twenties, I stayed with her while my mom went to Lancaster for a weekend. I told her we were going to eat the same things while I was there; I wasn't going to let her eat baby food. The first night I made myself a simple chili with ground beef, kidney beans, and tomatoes. I took out a portion for her before I added the seasonings, pureed it in the blender and fed it to her for dinner. Later, after we'd gone to bed, I heard her laughing in her room, which was next to mine. She rarely laughed. When she did, it was usually at something simple—a sneeze or some other unexpected loud noise. I got up to check on her and heard her passing gas. Each time she "tooted," she laughed. We both lay in our beds laughing, me until I cried. I still smile when I think about that night.

Kathy had to be monitored constantly and could never be left alone. She would sometimes grab hold of a crib slat or blanket and, because she couldn't let go, would scream bloody murder until one of us pried her fingers loose. It was terrifying to think that could happen with no one around to help. Someone in the family was always left behind with her except in the rare instance we took her with us, which was tough with seven others in the car.

We had a babysitter, Regina, who was more like a mother's helper, from the time I was small until I was in the second grade. She was very good with Kathy and often stayed with her when we went on day trips. We seldom went away overnight, but when we did, my dad's parents would stay with her. We all loved Kathy very much and never considered her a burden. She died of pneumonia in March of 1981 at the age of twenty-eight. We never thought of our family situation as special or different—but it was.

I was born May 22, 1956, when Kathy was nearly four. My mom had a couple of miscarriages between the two of us. She told me my dad was so happy when she became pregnant with me that he bought her a fur coat. My parents added four more children in the five years following; three boys in a row; Nick, Mark, and Paul, and then our baby sister, Joanna, who was born the day after my fifth birthday.

When I was four, we moved from our house on Main Street in Conemaugh to a home my dad had built about five miles away in Vinco. Vinco was "out in the country," and the new house sat in the middle of forty-five acres. There was much more room here; lots of outdoor space where our growing family could play, including a densely wooded area with plenty of trees to climb. The elementary school was half a mile from the house, close enough for us to walk, but we never did. My parents always drove us to and from school.

Weekday mornings were a madhouse once we were all in school. My dad used to say that breakfast at our house was a good example of why couples should use birth control. This from a man who would respond with "I have six, but I want six of each" when people would ask how many kids he had.

My mom was not a good cook. She was a very creative person, but she was so overwhelmed with all life had dealt her that she could only do what was absolutely necessary when it came to making meals for her family. She always made a delicious breakfast, though. We usually had eggs "sunny side up," toast (white Wonder Bread, of course), and bacon or sausages. Often she would serve sliced oranges, which I loved. We drank Ovaltine, orange juice, and whole milk—and we all drank coffee from the time we were very young. On weekends, we were allowed cereal. I remember Puffed Rice, Wheat Chex, Life, Trix, Cap'n Crunch, Froot Loops, and Cocoa Krispies.

When I started first grade, my mom usually packed a lunch for me in my red-plaid metal lunch box with its matching thermos. She made me a chipped ham sandwich, filled the thermos with Campbell's chicken noodle soup, and added a little bag of oyster crackers. I typically bought a carton of milk at school. Once more of us were in school, we were usually given money to buy lunch; it was easier on my mom. I believe it cost about thirty-five cents back then. We had the best school cafeteria at Vinco Elementary. Daisy Rose (that was her married name) was our school cook assisted by a couple of other older women who prepared delicious meals for us. One of my favorites was the ham, cabbage, and potato soup Daisy made—and I didn't even like cabbage. I've never had apple crisp as good as the one she made with a sweet, crisp, crunchy oatmeal topping. Tomato soup and grilled cheese sandwiches, chicken noodle soup, chili, spaghetti with meat sauce—everything was homemade and delicious.

Back at home, our evening meal was more often than not a TV dinner. Mom would pull five of the same meal out of the freezer—Morton's or Swanson's roast beef, Salisbury steak, fried chicken, sliced turkey or roast beef with gravy. I must admit that I liked them. Once in a while Mom would make creamed chipped beef or creamed "ring bologna" (more accurately called garlic bologna) over toast and served with mashed potatoes. Minute Rice was big at our house, too, with butter. We didn't always have salad; when we did, it was iceberg lettuce swimming in Italian or French dressing. My mother also had a fascination with Jell-o. I liked it, but over the years I grew to detest it because we had it so often. My mom's favorite way to prepare it was to add either canned fruit salad or mandarin oranges, but we had Jell-o hundreds of ways—or at least it seemed that way to me. My dad liked it with shredded cabbage and carrots. He called that "Spic and Span" Jell-o because it had the same color specks in it as the cleaning product with that name.

Mom sometimes made a four-ingredient chili, which was good. Her garlic bread, made with garlic powder and butter, was excellent. It was little wonder; she probably used half a pound of butter on a loaf of Italian bread. Weekend and summer lunches were usually sandwiches. Letizia's, the only grocery store in Vinco, had a deli filled with local meats and cheeses. We loved chipped ham, hard salami, and Longhorn and American cheeses.

If you're unfamiliar with chipped ham, it's a Western Pennsylvania specialty. A square loaf of ham parts sliced so thin you can see through them. It makes pretty, curly stacks of meat in a sandwich. My parents bought pounds and pounds of it every week. The local fire department, the Jackson Township Volunteer Fire Company, headquartered a half mile from our house, made delicious submarine sandwiches to raise money, which they delivered to our door every other Saturday for a dollar a piece. They were always a big hit with us kids.

Sundays we ate our main meal midday. We had baked chicken, ham, or roast beef, potatoes, and canned or frozen veggies. I think we had corn more than any other vegetable, followed by peas. We also got freshly baked baguettes from Letizia's on Sundays, which were a real treat. We ate them as soon as we got home, slathered with soft butter. For a doctor's family, it seems as though we ate an inordinately large amount of pretzels, potato chips, and crackers as snacks. Back then, the Charles Chips truck delivered snacks and cookies to the door. We would devour tins of their chocolate chip cookies after a long day of playing. Ice cream was our usual dessert, and there were always ice cream bars or popsicles in the fridge. We seldom had cake or pie, unless it was a special occasion. However, we did have Tastykake snack pies and cupcakes, which we consumed by the box. Crème filled chocolate cupcakes, delicate white cakes with coconut, and little rectangular fruit pies were often available at home and in our packed lunches for school.

My dad and his siblings had been brought up in the Russian Orthodox church, but we only went to church on Christmas and Easter as kids. Easter was great in the Russian church. My paternal grandmother, Mary, would make beautiful decorated eggs, called *pisanka* or *pisanki*, etched with hot wax in intricate designs and then dyed in deep, dark hues to accent the designs preserved under the wax. My dad's mother taught my mother this art, then my mom developed her own, more contemporary style of decorating eggs. She would do demonstrations for groups such as the PTA, and she was popular in our community over Easter. The eggs my grandmother made had hundreds of years of tradition behind them and were used to decorate the baskets of food the priest blessed after midnight mass. This meal was eaten early in the morning, at two or three a.m., after church to break the Lenten fast. My grandmother made homemade cheeses and bread for the basket, which also contained butter, horseradish, ham, and locally made *kolbassi*, a peppery smoked Polish pork sausage.

My dad's mother was the best cook in the family and made wonderful comfort foods—carbohydrate and fat-laden, of course. Our favorites were her homemade bread, pierogis, and fried pork chops. Pierogis are the eastern European version of ravioli. The dough is like noodle dough, with one less egg, according to Grandma Trahanovsky's recipe. Instead of Italian cheeses, pierogis are typically filled with cheddar cheese and mashed potatoes, sauerkraut, or prunes. My grandmother mostly made the cheese-and-potato-filled variety, which, once boiled, she tossed with chopped onions sautéed in oil, adding butter after the onions browned. Mark always requested *bobalka*, long snakelike ropes of the pierogi dough tossed with butter and onions. Grandma always made extras for him. She also made the best pork chops I've ever eaten, prepared like schnitzel. She pounded them oh-so-thin with a regular carpenter's hammer she kept in her kitchen drawer for that purpose, breaded them with crushed saltine crackers, then deep fried them in a cast-iron skillet in Mazola corn oil. She swore by Mazola. The pork chops were crisp and crunchy and simply out of this world. I can't imagine the amount of fat and calories in a big plate of those!

Grandma made her homemade bread without measuring anything, just as she made everything else—she said she baked "by feel." She mixed the ingredients in a big porcelain dishpan and worked them with her slender hands. As a child I was fascinated watching her cook and bake. She formed the dough into round loaves that she placed into ceramic mixing bowls. She then gently braided the remaining dough into long ropes and decorated the tops of the loaves with those. After rising, but before being placed in the hot oven, she brushed the bread with an "egg wash" (an egg and a little milk beaten together), which gave them a gorgeous golden crust. She rubbed the finished bread with a little Mazola to make them gleam. They were works of art. As kids we would tear off chunks of the fresh, warm bread and dip them into honey or soft butter. It was simply delicious.

On holidays or when she had company, which was often, the table in her sitting room was laden with plates of pierogis, pork chops, loaves of homemade bread and cheeses, platters of sliced baked ham, *halupki* (cabbage rolls stuffed with ground meat and rice in a tomato sauce), *kolbassi*, potato salad and various baked goods. She frequently had a pot of beef stock simmering on the stove and homemade egg noodles in the fridge. When you wanted soup, you would grab a handful of noodles and put them in a bowl. Grandma would then ladle the steaming hot broth with big chunks of beef and vegetables over the top. If anyone ever left my grandparent's home hungry, it was his or her own fault. Her sitting room had strands of mushrooms suspended along the walls in some stage of the drying process most all year round. She picked wild mushrooms from the fields near our home in Vinco when I was a child, but later on she bought them at the market. She used a needle and thread to string them into garlands and roped them around their large coal stove to dry, and years later, around the coal furnace. She used the dried mushrooms to make a rich mushroom gravy.

She made poppy-seed rolls and walnut rolls that were fantastic. A delicate spice cake and rustic apple pies and apple dumplings, Grandpap's favorite, were the only other desserts I recall. If we were hungry late in the evening, she'd tear slices of bread into chunks in a cereal bowl, top them with hot milk and sprinkle them with sugar. This infuriated my dad, who was not a fan of sugar, but to us "bread and milk" was heavenly. Her house also was the only place we were allowed to have soda, which during my childhood was a treat, not a beverage. Grandma and Grandpap kept glass bottles of grape and orange Nehi as well as root beer and cream soda in the crisper drawer of the Frigidaire. My dad's opinion of soda was that it would "rot your kidneys." To this day I'm not a soda drinker and have it only a few times a year, usually 7Up or root beer.

When I was seven my parents built a swimming pool. We were one of the first families in Vinco to have an inground pool, and it was a magnet for friends and family. We had lots of company, thanks to the pool; we all loved it. Every free moment all summer, every summer was spent in that pool for the rest of our childhood. We went to bed with our swimsuits on as soon as school let out in June so we wouldn't miss a moment in the pool.

We became friends with two older cousins, Harry and Tommy, from the Westmont area of Johnstown. The would come to swim, bringing big plastic jugs of Lance's peanut butter crackers and cheese and crackers for us to snack on. When it was too cold to swim (nearly nine months of the year), we climbed trees, caught crayfish and "minnies" (minnows) in the stream that ran through our property, or built make-believe forts in the woods. My mom would shoo us out of the house and we were happy to go. We were a very active bunch. We all tried to keep up with one another—no one wanted to be the slacker of the group and get left out. We played outside pretty much from morning to night when we weren't in school.

Both of my parents were overweight during our school years; my mom was obese. She was five foot three and weighed at least 250 pounds throughout our childhood. My youngest brother Paul and I were the first of the kids to have issues with our weight. My siblings and I have all struggled with our weight at some point—except for Mark, who has always stayed physically active and exercises great restraint in eating.

When I hit puberty at age eleven, I was five feet tall and weighed a hundred pounds. I grew four inches and gained twenty pounds the following year. I went from being very active to feeling awkward about the changes taking place in my body. I was confused by what was happening and couldn't control any of it. No one ever prepared me for getting my period. When I was in the fifth grade, I saw blood on my underwear one morning and thought I must be dying. I had heard my dad talk about cancer, and I figured that was what was wrong with me. I was too afraid to tell anyone.

My mom found my underwear when she was doing the laundry. She came to school, had me taken out of class, and took me home to change my clothes, making me feel even more embarrassed and ashamed. One night soon after, she gave me a book, *What Teenagers Want to Know,* so I could learn about sex and the changes taking place in my body. I think that book was meant as a tool to help parents discuss sex with their children, not for an eleven-year-old to figure out on her own. I was appropriately disgusted by almost everything in the book.

For the next several years, I suffered with a poor self-image. I could no longer run and jump and play with my three younger brothers or swim when I had my period. I felt different and left out. Having to be out of the pool for several days every month was devastating. I wasn't introduced to tampons until years later. I had to wear a "sanitary napkin" hooked in the front and back to an elastic "belt" worn under my underwear. It was indescribably awful. God bless the person who invented pads that stick to underwear.

I remember going clothes shopping for school later that same year and wanting a certain outfit. It was a red plaid jumper with a skirt that flared out when I twirled around. I loved it. In the dressing room, my mom told me I could get it, but I had to promise to lose weight. I said I would so I could get the dress, but wondered how I was supposed to lose weight when she was the one preparing my meals.

I had always loved reading. The first day of fourth grade, I opened my geography book to see a young African native. The textbook was full of stories about children all over the world—what a wonderful way to learn! I couldn't wait to read all about the kids and learn about where they lived. Now I could retreat from my world into the pages of books, which transported me from the tiny village of Vinco to wonderful new places. I could taste the homemade cheese Heidi's grandfather spread on freshly baked bread and see the sparkling fresh snow in the Swiss Alps through her eyes. I raced to fires in a horse-drawn wagon in *Blitz, the Story of a Horse*. I devoured all of Marguerite Henry's books after reading *Misty of Chincoteague*. I read *Black Beauty, My Friend Flicka*, and any book about horses I could get my hands on. Agatha Christie, Ellery Queen, Annette Funicello, and I all solved mysteries together. The bookmobile visited our elementary school every week or so, and I loaded up with new books each time. I brought my Scholastic books flyer home each month with a dozen books checked off. My mom told me I could only get five or six at a time. I couldn't wait to go to school the day the order was delivered. I owe my excellent spelling skills and vocabulary to the many books I read during my elementary school days.

Eating was the one thing in addition to reading that made me feel better. By the time I was a freshman in high school, I weighed 140 pounds. My classmates nicknamed me "Maya" in reference to an elephant on the popular television show *George of the Jungle*. I hated the nickname, obviously. In hindsight, I wasn't obese. I suppose I attracted the comments because I was so uncomfortable in my own skin.

CHAPTER THREE

Next Steps

In the five months following the AON climb, I train with one goal in mind: to improve my time in my second competitive climb. I want to lose weight, of course, but that will be a fringe benefit of getting into better shape. I'm tired of dieting only to lose weight and not necessarily become more fit. I prefer to push myself physically and see how that works. I pass a parking structure on my walks, and I begin doing flights of stairs there several days a week. There are eight flights of eight stairs each, sixty-four steps in one trip up the garage stairwell. I start by doing three sets and add one more each visit until I'm doing ten, twelve, and then fourteen or more sets. It's an excruciating workout. My lungs and quads burn each time I make a trip up the stairwell.

There is an ongoing discussion among stair climbers about the misuse of the words *flight* and *floor*. Most climbers agree that there are usually two flights of stairs between floors, so it is inappropriate to refer to the two sets as a flight. Therefore I use the word *flight* to describe a set of stairs. A floor may have one, two, or more flights. In the parking garage where I currently train, there are five floors, each with two flights between floors; so ten flights of ten steps each. A nine-story interior stairwell where I practice has twenty-five flights of between eight and twelve stairs each, totaling two hundred-fifty stairs.

I like to go the parking garage early in the morning when it's cool and quiet and there's no one else around. I catch my breath as much as possible in the elevator between ascents. The payoff is feeling like there's nothing I can't conquer when I'm done. Running stairs is a fast, effective cardio workout; it jump-starts the heart rate and keeps it pumping for the remainder of the workout. I always take the elevator down (when there's one available); it's easier on the knees.

Veteran climber Henry Wigglesworth is an inspiration to me and many other climbers and a legend in the climbing community. He enjoys stair workouts because you get "so much bang for your buck." Before his first climb, Henry would go for runs in his hometown of in Seattle with his infant daughter in a carrier on his back. When he added a nearby set of stairs on a steep neighborhood street to his route, he was surprised at how much harder it was than running. A friend invited him to do Seattle's Big Climb. The Big Climb in the Columbia Tower is the largest climb in North America, limited to the first *six thousand* registrants. He did better than he thought, but he knew he could be faster with more training, so he trained hard and won the Big Climb three years later.

Henry has a unique style: he races barefoot. He says climbing is "gentle on feet"—there's no impact on the feet like in running, no support needed. I ask Henry if he's ever stepped in anything sticky, and so far he hasn't, but that may be because he's usually at the front of the pack as an elite.

Henry also set a record of sorts one year when he did the Big Climb as part of a relay team. He paid for multiple entries so he could climb it more than once. Henry's time was better than any of his team members the first time up. And the second time. And the third time! The top three finishers on his team were all Henry. It looked like a typo when the results were posted. The last time Henry participated in the Big Climb, he did it seven times.

The Columbia Tower is the setting for one scene in the David Guterson's novel *The Others*. A character in a scene mentions the Big Climb and that "a guy named Wigglesworth won it in 2008 with a time of 8:07." Henry is still delighted when friends call to tell him they came upon his name while reading the book.

Most people, however, say they've never heard of competitive stair climbing when I mention my sport. Stair climbing has humble roots in the U.S. It began in New York City when a group of nine men decided in the late 1970s to climb the stairwells in tall buildings for exercise rather than brave the winter weather to run. As is the case with most sports, they tried to out-do one another—and, voilà, a new sport was born.

The second comment I get from people when I bring up climbing is typically, "Isn't that hard on your knees?" Climbing stairs is not hard on the knees, but running down stairs is. Over time, the impact of weight bearing down on the knees can cause damage. Running up or down stairs may cause issues for those with existing knee problems, however.

I had been taking daily walks on the beach since committing to my first climb, and now I begin running a few blocks during those walks to help with my stamina and learn to control my breathing. I had tried running in the past, first when I was a teenager and again in 2003, but I could never make it more than a few blocks; I couldn't breathe and would have to stop. Stair climbing has pushed me beyond that point, so now I work on building up the distances I run each week on the sand. I run four blocks, then walk four, off and on for a mile or so. I move to the pavement and work my way up to a mile and a half, alternating running with walking. In the five months between the two climbs, I'm not yet brave enough to step on a scale, but I know I'm still around 220 pounds. I am, however, firming and shaping my body and building muscle. My clothes are getting looser, so I know that what I'm doing is moving me in the right direction.

Come September, I feel fitter than I did in April. I've climbed many thousands of steps in preparation for the Ketchum Downtown Stair Climb for Los Angeles. The climb is held each September in the U.S. Bank Tower (originally called the Library Tower), the tallest building in California, the tallest office building west of the Mississippi, and currently the sixty-fifth tallest building in the world. Funds raised for this climb go to the Ketchum Downtown YMCA. The Y coordinates the climb and has been doing so for more than twenty years. In spite of that, climbers refer to this event as the U.S. Bank Climb, which I'm sure the Y is not crazy about. "The Y Climb" sounds too much like "The Why Climb."

As with my first climb, the start here is outside at the base of the building. A DJ plays very loud music and there are large digital time displays at the start. Water jugs and small paper cups are nearby, so I have a last-minute sip. I line up with the other female 50–59 AG participants and soon get sent inside. I trip on the second flight and nearly fall. My mind is racing ahead of my feet. *Slow down, take it easy,* I tell myself. It's a warm day and very hot in the stairwell. I wish I were thin enough to race in just a sports bra like some of the other women. There is a station set up with chairs, cold towels, and water toward the top of the building in an area off one of the landings. A volunteer looks at me with concern and asks if I'd like to rest for a moment. I can feel that my face is hot and red, so I sit down, press the cool cloth on my neck and face, have a sip of water, then hit the stairs again. The climb is excruciatingly hard, but I make it to the top one step at a time.

As a result of the work I've invested in preparing for today, I am able to trim my time to just over thirty minutes. I finish almost four minutes faster than at AON, even though the building has 1,679 stairs and—at seventy-five stories—is twelve stories taller.

I am so happy! I have never worked toward an athletic goal before, and I am extremely pleased with the results. I am even more driven now to excel in my second trip up the AON Building in April, and I have almost seven months to train.

Mark whizzed up the tower in 12:03, finishing third overall. My boss Craig's time did not show in the results. For this race, we had to affix a timing strip to our shoe. The strips are light, convenient, and disposable. They have an adhesive backing; each strip sticks to itself when fed through shoelaces. Never having used one before, when I applied Craig's, I crimped it and it didn't register his time. Thankfully, he's a good sport or else I might be unemployed. Craig and I had carpooled to the race, and I tell him on the way home that I plan on training hard for the next AON climb. I say, "Can you imagine how much faster I could be if I lost twenty pounds before the next climb?"

By the April 2009 AON climb, I *am* more than twenty pounds lighter. In addition to walking and riding my bike regularly, I've been climbing thousands of stairs a week to better my time and increase my fitness and lung capacity. I cut my time on that climb from over thirty-four minutes to just over twenty. Again, I am thrilled with my progress. I keep up my training in preparation for the 2009 U.S. Bank Climb in September.

My second trip up the U.S. Bank building does not show as much improvement, however. This is my first disappointing climb. Despite losing more weight and training hard, it takes me 30:55 to finish—thirty seconds slower than the 2008 climb. I didn't sleep well the night before, but it's hard to know why I was slower. Mark reminds me that, in a seventy-five-story building, being slower by one second per floor means it will take 1:15 longer to get to the top. Craig finishes in a respectable time of 19:58. Mark shows everyone up with a time of 11:58 and, out of 335 racers, is the overall winner of the open competition at the age of fifty. He's unbelievable.

This climb has the best motto of all the competitions as far as I'm concerned. Climbers look forward to getting a new T-shirt each year with "Elevators Are for Wimps" emblazoned across the front. I love wearing mine to exercise outdoors; I get lots of smiles from passersby. Organizers took some flack for the slogan; critics deemed it offensive to handicapped people.

At the time, a member of the YMCA had lost a leg as a result of a car accident. YMCA officials asked her if she was offended by the "Elevators Are for Wimps" slogan. She was not. She expressed an interest in stair climbing, so the Y volunteered to help her train, and she did the climb in 2007. She said she wanted to inspire her grandchildren. One of her grandchildren did the 2013 climb. Grandma was there at the finish, but she got to the top that time via the elevator.

CHAPTER FOUR

Tiptoeing

Something that took my family years to come to terms with, and something we still deal with today, was the fact that my dad was an alcoholic. Because of my dad's position in the community, we dared not share this shameful secret. No one who hasn't lived with an alcoholic parent can imagine the utter devastation an alcoholic parent wreaks on a family. My dad never drank socially; he was a binge drinker. Once he had a drink, he didn't stop until he ran out of alcohol. In our house, that's when the horror began. My dad would plead with my mom to go out and get him more liquor. If she didn't, which was always, he would get violent and call her curse words I have never heard another human being utter to this day. He would never hit or punch her, but he would bully her, pinning her against the wall and smashing things. We didn't have a door in our home that hadn't been broken down. He would scream, yell, threaten, and stomp through the house for hours on end. One night, I stood barefoot in the snow wearing only my nightgown, screaming to create a distraction so my parents would stop fighting. It didn't work.

Our home life was a nightmare when he drank. A neighbor told me many years later that she could hear us screaming, and it broke her heart. Dad would take to a couch in the cellar when he was finally exhausted and convinced that he wasn't getting any more booze, and moan and cry endlessly until he fell asleep. If you think waking a sleeping baby is rough, the fallout from waking a drunken rage-aholic who is out of booze is unimaginable. We tiptoed around to avoid waking my dad when he was in this state so all hell wouldn't break loose all over again.

Many times at this point my mom would pack us up in the car and take us to stay at a motel. At times she would drive us to her parents' home in Lancaster. When we got there, we had to pretend that everything was okay, but it was far from it. Once we drove for four hours to within a few miles of my grandparents' home, and my mom decided to stay in a motel instead. She didn't want to explain why we were showing up out of the blue so late at night. We all had to sleep in our clothes because we didn't have time to pack anything when we left. We turned around and drove nearly two hundred miles back home the next morning without ever telling our grandparents we were there. Episodes like this during my childhood led me to have control and trust issues later in life.

Sometimes we went away without Kathy; my mom's logic was that my dad would sober up if he had to take care of her. Thank God, he always did. That was the situation the day President Kennedy was assassinated. I was in second grade, my dad was drunk, and we left to go to Lancaster. We stopped at a roadside diner for a meal on the way. Our waitress said the president had been shot in Dallas and later told us he had died, so we turned around and went home. My mom thought that news would sober my dad up, and it did. Until I was an adult, when people discussed where they were when they heard the news that President Kennedy was shot, I could never tell the truth about where I was. I had to tell them what was written on the excuse my mom sent with me when I returned to school. I was absent because I had "intestinal influenza." At some point that year, my teacher commented that I certainly had intestinal influenza a lot.

I wanted to tell her to talk to my mother about that, but as usual, I had to remain silent. I remember being of elementary school age and having to pee during the night or get a drink of water. I would slink down the hallway one step at a time careful not to make the floor creak so as not to wake and anger my dad. I flattened myself against the wall and sidestepped along the hallway, pretending that I was a secret agent trying to break into our house undetected. I can't imagine putting a child through such an ordeal to satisfy a basic need. If he had been drinking and heard any of us up and about, my dad would bellow, "Who's up? What are you doing?" and fly into a rage.

When he wasn't drinking, he was an entirely different person, like Dr. Jekyll and Mr. Hyde. He'd get up with us during the night, tell stories, and make us scrambled eggs with fried strips of ham or Mexicorn (corn with diced peppers). I don't know why he added the corn, but he sure liked that combination.

One year for his birthday when I was about eight or nine, my mom sent us into Letizia's, the little local market, to get him a cake before he came home from the office. We bought a little yellow premade boxed cake with chocolate icing and took it home to put candles in it. We lined up and surprised him with it when he walked in the door. The surprise was on us, however. He flew into a rage, took it to the kitchen, shoved it down the garbage disposal, and ground it up. He yelled, screamed, and took a bottle of Scotch to his room—and that was the beginning of another binge-drinking event in my childhood. It may have been his fortieth birthday, and, as an adult, I can appreciate that he might have been disappointed that my mom hadn't made more of an effort, but his outburst was devastating to five small children lined up with a gift for their dad. It was such a selfish act. We grew up in a very isolated existence; my brothers and sister and I stuck together like glue, because my mom told us, "You can never trust your friends, only your family."

For our birthdays we got cake and ice cream for dessert after our evening meal. Not one of us ever got to invite a friend to celebrate a birthday during our childhood. We couldn't risk making a plan to have someone come to our house in case my dad would get drunk. I was astonished at the huge birthday celebrations my daughter's friends had as kids, and I made sure my daughter always had a party with a theme and friends from the time she was in kindergarten. It was much different for the five of us. None of us ever was allowed to have a friend sleep overnight for the same reason. Every once in a while, one of us would ask if we could invite a friend over, and Mom would answer with, "What if your dad gets drunk?" That was the end of that.

It was very confusing to hear people talk about how wonderful my dad was, especially my mom, all the while knowing what a monster he was when he was drunk. We never knew which dad we would have from day to day. When he was sober, my dad was honestly the best dad in the world. I cannot imagine having a better dad during those times. He was fun and imaginative. When I was in first grade, he built us an A-frame playhouse that we practically lived in all summer. Several years later, he topped that with a two-story playhouse we called the "tree house," even though there was no tree involved in the structure of the building. It had Anderson windows that opened, insulation, and a gabled roof. He built us a wooden bridge that crossed the small stream that ran through our property. We spent countless hours playing "Billy Goats Gruff" on that little bridge. He used to take us on "jungle tours" through tall grass on the property in our Jeep, fondly named Hercules. My brothers ate it up. I was afraid and hung on for dear life, fearing we would roll over at any moment. One beautiful summer evening, he mowed the field across from our house into a maze. We ran through the paths cut into the freshly cut grass until we couldn't run any more.

In 1967 my dad took us on a cross-country road trip for his brother Walter's wedding in Iowa. We drove to Colorado after the wedding and saw the Rocky Mountains for the first time. When he was sober we took shorter road trips almost every weekend, visiting Bedford, Somerset, Altoona, Indiana, Niagara Falls, Luray Caverns in Virginia, and the Poconos. My dad was a steam engine nut. We rode every steam locomotive within a two hundred-mile radius of our home.

All these road trips involved eating along the way at wonderful diners and local eateries. We had fried clams and coffee ice cream at Howard Johnson's, hot turkey and hot roast beef sandwiches with mashed potatoes and gravy at Dave's Dream in Hollidaysburg. We ate chicken and waffles (with more gravy), steamed clams, burgers and shakes, Wing Dings (chicken wings) at Nagle's in Ebensburg, French fries, ice-cream cones and sundaes, doughnuts and much, much more. We each got a postcard from Howard Johnson's before our birthdays and sometimes got to go there for a special birthday dinner. I always ordered the beef burgundy and couldn't wait for the birthday cake. They served a coconut cake (still my favorite kind of cake) on a little spinning musical cake stand.

One afternoon shortly before Christmas 1971, during my sophomore year of high school, my dad called out to me for help. He had been on a bender for days, and now was lying drunk on my parent's bedroom floor. He asked for a tissue, and I saw that he was spitting up blood. He told me not to tell my mom. Later that evening my mom was on the phone with my dad's Uncle Harry, also a doctor. My mom had been talking to Uncle Harry about my dad's condition. He had been seeing things—rats and spiders climbing up the walls, for example, which typically was a symptom of delirium tremens. Harry told my mom to call him if he started spitting up blood. When I told my mom that he was, Harry told her to call an ambulance and get him to the hospital. Dad screamed and yelled and cried when the paramedics arrived, saying if he was going to die, he wanted to die at home. It was awful; I hid outside on the side of the house when they took him away. Once in the hospital, his condition worsened. He had diabetes and cirrhosis of the liver. He went into a coma and spent weeks in ICU. He was in critical condition and was given the last rights of the church.

During this same time, Kathy suffered a broken leg. Her thighbone snapped while my mom was feeding her one evening. She had to have surgery to repair the bone and was placed in a room at the opposite end of the ICU where my dad was. To everyone's surprise, my dad, who was in and out of consciousness, asked his nurse one day if someone would give Kathy some water because she was thirsty—he recognized her cry even though he was unaware she was even in the hospital. By the end of January, he improved and was moved out of ICU.

We had just gotten home from school on February 10, 1972, when my mom got a call from Harry saying we should come to the hospital right away. My dad had suffered a stroke as a result of his high blood pressure. Nick and my mom and I went; Mark, Paul, and Joanna stayed at home with Kathy. When we got to the room, my dad looked like he was asleep. We stayed for a few minutes, and then Harry asked us to step outside into a small waiting area. He joined us after a few minutes and said something to my mom. I thought Uncle Harry said, "He's coming along," but he actually had said, "He's gone." All I remember is Harry sighing and leaning back into the wall. I felt as though a sharp sword had sliced me through from the top of my head to the bottom of my feet.

My dad's death was a crushing blow. Despite everything, I adored him. I was very distant from my mom and only wanted to be with him. Everything he did was so much more interesting than staying home to clean and do laundry like my mother. He was powerful and well liked as well as being a brilliant diagnostician. He mostly did tonsillectomies, gall bladder surgeries and appendectomies, but many doctors in the area called him when they were stumped on a case, and my dad would give them his opinion.

He was on the phone one day with an MD from Johnstown who asked if he'd heard that another local doctor had been ill. "Dr. A" started describing to my dad what "Dr. B's" symptoms were, and my dad said it sounded like Dr. B had tuberculosis of the brain. Dr. A went silent, then told my dad that Dr. B had been to "every doctor in town" and in Pittsburgh and had ended up at the Cleveland Clinic for testing before anyone came up with that diagnosis. My dad had correctly diagnosed Dr. B without ever laying eyes on him. TV's Dr. House reminds me of my dad: brilliant and volatile. When he died I felt lost and hopeless; the most important person in my world was gone.

I learned the most important lesson in my life the day of my dad's funeral. He was buried in his best suit, a kind of gold tweed pattern— pretty flashy for my dad. I remember him coming home when he bought it and being so pleased with himself. All of his other suits were plain black, gray, or blue; this one was special, stylish. As they lowered his coffin into the ground, I thought about what mattered in life. Not that suit, not his fancy cars, not our house or our pool. I realized that the only thing that counted for anything, the only thing that lasted beyond the grave, were the relationships he had with the people in his life.

I eventually ended up having a good relationship with my mother, but at the time, I thought God had made one huge mistake in taking my dad away from us. To make matters even worse, Dad didn't believe in investing in life insurance. He thought he would live forever (that God complex again). He left us with $30,000 in life insurance in 1972. My mom had never worked outside the home or dealt with the family budget; my dad had controlled everything. She asked Uncle Harry, a seasoned investor, to invest the money so she would have an income. He invested it wisely, but my mom cashed in stocks every time she needed money and depleted the account within a few years. By the time I started college, our family was pretty much broke.

Coming from a tumultuous background like mine created deeply rooted issues that plagued me and led to a life of overindulgence. I sought comfort in food and, later on, alcohol and tobacco.

CHAPTER FIVE

Formative Steps

My first job was at the Dairy Queen while I was high school. My friend Tera worked there and helped me get the job. We were paid $1.10 per hour, half the minimum wage, and got to make all the items we served. I loved it! Making parfaits, shakes, sundaes, and banana splits tapped into my creative nature and was a lot like playing restaurant at home, which we did as kids—only better, of course, because all the equipment and the money was real. I worked there for about a year and didn't work again until I dropped out of college in 1974.

I wanted to go to school to become a veterinarian. I had wanted to be a vet since I was a little girl because I've always loved animals. I fed, bathed, and cared for my family's two dogs, Knish and Hesse, from the time I was in the first grade. It was Hesse, the German Shepherd we got for Christmas in 1963, who I ran to for comfort when my dad died. It was a freezing cold February night, but I ran outside to grieve with Hesse as soon as we got home from the hospital. Hesse sat in silence with my arms wrapped around him as I cried until I couldn't cry anymore. He never moved a muscle. He was my angel; I loved him so much. He lived to be about sixteen years old.

I had good grades throughout my school years and graduated in the top 20 percent of my class. My mom thought that if I was going to invest so much time getting a doctorate, I should become a "people doctor," not "waste" years of education on animals. I wanted to go to Franklin and Marshall College in Lancaster and live with my grandmother. My mom thought I should go to the University of Pittsburgh and live in a dorm. She was afraid my grandmother would die and disrupt my education. Looking back I think I wanted a mother figure, someone who would take care of me. We split the difference.

I went to Pittsburgh as a biology/premed major and got an apartment with a girl from Vinco who I'd known since second grade. This ended up being a terrible idea. My roommate was an only child; she had money and was a drinker and loved to party. I was always broke, and I was easily coerced into partying and drinking to excess with her and her friends. All that fun lasted for one semester. My grades were awful, and I felt lost and alone, so I quit school and moved back home. The truth was I hadn't been given the tools I needed to succeed on my own; I wasn't mature enough. Once I was living back at my mom's house, I needed money for food and gas, so I got a job at McDonald's on Main Street in downtown Johnstown.

For all the grief McDonald's takes about its food, this job provided the best possible training I could have gotten for my future career in the food service industry. The owner's name was Ron, as in Ronald McDonald, which Mark thought was hilarious. Ron not-McDonald trained us to always think from the customer's point of view. If we dropped a bunch of straws on the floor, they were tossed in the trash if it happened in front of a customer. Even though they were individually wrapped, the customer might perceive that we were giving them something dirty because it had been on the floor. All our bills had to face the same way in the cash drawer. The restaurant was immaculate, the staff happy and professional.

Ron worked the line and expedited the food during the busy lunch rush. He was an excellent restaurateur. I learned many good things in the brief time I spent there, lessons I took with me to future jobs. While I was still working at Micky D's, my mom and I ate out one night in 1974 to the Encore Restaurant and Lounge in the Richland Mall. The Richland Mall was the area's newest and largest shopping mall at the time, located near the Cambria County Airport. My parents had frequented the owners' previous restaurant, Campanella's, since I was an infant. Rose Campanella, the owner, came to our table and reminisced about carrying me around the kitchen as a baby. She said I should come work for her, so I did. From 1975 to 2003, I worked in restaurants. For twenty of those years, I was a waitress.

I started as a bus girl and was promoted to waitress as soon as I figured out how things worked. The Encore's two chefs were Jim Loveridge and Frank Lombardo, both of who later would open their own very successful restaurants in Johnstown. The food was fantastic. In 1975 the Encore featured a $4.95 "all you can eat" seafood buffet on Friday nights. Customers lined up around the outside of the mall waiting to get in. The buffet featured all freshly prepared items; clam chowder, baked and deep fried scallops, broiled and breaded fried haddock and cod, stuffed clams, fried shrimp, steamed shrimp, shrimp creole, rice, macaroni and cheese, salads, and many other items I can't remember. The only item we never ran out of was shrimp creole. We were allowed to eat what was left at the end of the night, including the rice and all the salad items. I've never eaten shrimp creole since. We ran at top speed from the time we started our shift around four in the afternoon until late at night. What a training experience that was!

As a rookie I was assigned to a huge section at the back of the restaurant. It served as the cocktail lounge after hours and was packed with tables. The more experienced girls, Janice and Minnie, got the better sections with fewer tables. Guests at those tables were regulars who typically drank wine and cocktails and ordered higher priced items, such as steak and lobster, off the regular menu. Back in the lounge where I was, things were "turn and burn." As soon as guests were seated, I took their beverage order, set them loose on the buffet, and stayed busy clearing empty dishes and refilling water glasses and coffee cups as fast as possible for the rest of the night.

I soon adapted to the life of a waitress. They're referred to as "servers" these days, but in the Johnstown area in the seventies, there were no waiters, only waitresses. Men were bartenders or worked in the kitchen. Waitresses wore white uniforms and white shoes and were supposed to wear hairnets. We hated them for reasons of vanity but kept them in our pockets in case health inspectors showed up. If they did, we had to quickly put one over our hair. We were tipped almost exclusively in cash; very few people charged their meals unless they needed a record for business purposes. At the end of the day, we walked out with wads of cash. I don't remember the exact amount I made back then, but I took home at least forty or fifty dollars per shift and sometimes much more, which was good money at the time.

Even before I turned twenty-one, we would go out drinking after work. For me going out was what made going to work worthwhile. I was the youngest of the servers at the Encore by far and didn't get carded since everyone else was older. We drank at local bars, met guys, danced, and generally had a blast. Waitresses are "people persons" and boy, do they know how to have fun! The other waitresses all smoked, so I started smoking, too. My memories of those days are full of laughter and listening to story after story. Many times, we'd go out to dinner before going to a bar if we were finished with work early enough.

Restaurants have different policies about feeding their employees. Most will allow employees to have soup, salad, and bread or rolls free of charge and offer a limited number of items at cost for their employees. If you work in one restaurant long enough, that gets boring fast, and if you go out drinking after, you need food to keep you going. We ate many a

Grand Slam at Denny's after two o'clock in the morning when the bars closed or enjoyed omelets and hot dogs at Coney Island downtown. When I think of all the money I spent on cigarettes and alcohol in my twenties, it makes me sick, but we sure had fun while it lasted.

The running around at work, dancing afterward, and a youthful metabolism helped keep the extra pounds off for a while, but my weight eventually caught up with me. I fell into a very bad routine that led me down a path of promiscuity and alcohol abuse. If things didn't go my way, which they often didn't, I drank to make myself feel better. This was acceptable behavior in my peer group and went unchecked for many years.

My sex education came courtesy of *Cosmopolitan* magazine, which I started reading when I was sixteen. Cosmo made it seem as though everyone was having great sex all the time, and I felt left out. I also thought that sex would make me feel complete and fill the emptiness I felt inside. All I wanted was for someone to love me, and at that point in my life, it seemed like sex was the way to get it. I wanted to "save myself" for marriage, but at the age of twenty-two, I gave up. I had already begun looking for love in all the wrong places, as the song goes, and had started going home with guys I met in bars. Almost without exception, these turned out to be one-night stands, which taught me the hard way that sex and love are two totally different things.

This lifestyle led me to being overweight and unhealthy. I stayed out late drinking and never exercised—work was my exercise. I slept from two, three, or four o'clock in the morning until eleven the next morning. I never ate breakfast; I just drank lots of coffee or black tea and then ate something before I went to work for the evening. I'm certain that most of my calories during those years were consumed in liquid form. I was fortunate that constantly being on my feet, walking and shuttling food for eight or more hours a day, kept me somewhat fit.

Letting go of food as a friend and source of happiness and solace was a feat I thought impossible until 2010.

CHAPTER SIX

Faster Steps

After the disappointing race at U.S. Bank in 2009, I'm determined to train even harder for the 2010 AON climb. I run more and more stairs and, thanks in part to a "Body & Soul" program at my church, I lose another thirty pounds by April 2010. I do very well my third time up this building; my time is 16:47—less than half the 34:14 time of my first AON climb two years earlier. I am amazed and encouraged that once again my hard work has paid off.

I'm not at all happy when I see the overall results, though. Craig and I always have a little office rivalry about who will beat whom. He has had a better time than mine on every climb we've done so far, and in this race has beaten me by just three seconds with a time of 16:44. Jeannie Rasmussen places third in our AG and nudges me out of a medal by two seconds. Mark recruited Jeannie, a client of his, into the sport. She is a runner and has medaled in numerous 5ks, which carries over well to this climb, her first.

I had paused to grab a cup of water on the trip up, and I feel as though that probably cost me third place and the loss to Craig. I'd learned since my first race to hydrate well in the days leading up to a race to prevent extreme thirst during the climb. I drank as much water as I could in the three days preceding this event, but nerves made my mouth dry and I had to have that water. I vow to never again stop for a drink. This will be the last race when Craig's time is better than mine.

I continue to train hard. I don't want to have another disappointing race at U.S. Bank. I begin running regularly in May. My daughter Ariana, now twenty-two, had competed in track and cross-country in high school and offers to help me train. We have a great relationship and she's a sweet kid, but she turns out to be quite the taskmaster as a coach. At first, we run about half a mile, stop to stretch, then run back home. I beg her to let me stop along the way. I tell her I'm going to pass out; I have a side cramp; I can't breathe. She tells me to shut up and keep running. I plead with her and swear I can't take one more step, but she urges me on. There's one traffic light on the way home; I pray the entire leg back, "Please give me a red light, Lord!" Sometimes I get it and can catch my breath; other times, I do not. We add more distance every week. I eventually build up my stamina and am able to run three miles without stopping by the end of summer. I'm on my own at this point, because Ariana actually hates running and doesn't run regularly.

I establish a routine of running an average of five mornings a week. I alternate between three routes: the first one flat on the beachfront boardwalk, the second a two-mile loop that includes a steep grade on the first half of the route. The third route is just under three miles round trip, but mostly all flat. I begin by running every other morning but find myself making excuses to stay in bed, telling myself I'll make up for it the next day. I then feel lousy and beat my self up emotionally for being a slacker the rest of the day. It's not worth the few extra minutes of sleep. I need to go to bed earlier.

I switch to running Tuesday through Saturday to coincide with my work schedule and take Sunday and Monday off. This works better for me— I have to get up early anyway. I start work at 8:45 a.m., so I get up at 6:15 instead of 6:45 to fit in a run. Sometimes I run half a mile to my favorite parking garage, do several hundred stairs, and then run back home. I am easily bored, so varied routines keep me from getting discouraged. My iPod is the best running tool ever, though. The best inspiration for me when running or climbing is music, mainly rock and roll. I run to Blondie, Katy Perry, the Eurythmics, Springsteen, Aretha, the Stones, and Prince. I don't think I could run half a mile without my music. Okay, I could, but I'd be miserable.

I hate running, too. After years of running hundreds and hundreds of miles and even completing two 5ks, I still go to bed dreading having to run the next morning. I procrastinate before runs and have to do positive self-talk to get myself out the door. For the first several blocks, I'm fine. After that, every step and each breath is a chore and so boring. I listen to music, pray, and look at the scenery to keep my mind off the drudgery. I tell myself that running is preferable to fighting cancer or suffering loss like many of my friends have had to do. When I finish, I feel fantastic, thankfully, because that's my motivation to get up the next morning and do it again.

By September, I peel off another forty pounds by sticking to my eating plan and staying active. I'm now more than eighty pounds lighter than the day of my first climb. I have had dogs my whole life, so all I can picture is the me I am today carrying bags of dog food on that first climb. No wonder it took me over half an hour! There's no way I would do the U.S. Bank race today carrying a fifty pound, twenty-five pound, and five pound bag of dog food strapped to my back. It would be ridiculous, but that's how much additional weight I carried on my first climb. Even the very fit "High Rise Heroes"—firefighters who climb wearing sixty pounds of gear—struggle on their way to the top. I am so grateful to be fit and trim now.

While we're hanging out waiting to line up for the 2010 U.S. Bank Climb in late September, someone asks Mark how he got into stair climbing. He says it's actually because of Ariana. I can't imagine what he means—Ariana and I learned about stair climbing from Mark. He explains that he had met Tim Van Orden, from runningraw.com, at a race at Loyola Marymount University in May of 2007. Ariana was a freshman at LMU and had invited Mark to do a 5k with her there. Mark struck up a conversation with Tim after the race and mentioned that he had bad knees. Tim said he should try a sport with less impact on the knees and told him about competitive stair climbing. Mark made his first climb at U.S. Bank that September.

Because of the large number of climbers (nearly two thousand including firefighters) registered this year, we don't take off until about 8:00 p.m. I'm yawning by the time my age group begins lining up at the start. I feel as though my adrenaline has bottomed out, and I'm honestly ready to go home and go to bed.

When I finally get into the stairwell, my trip up is hot and sweaty but uneventful, aside from this being the only race during which Mark passes me. Mark starts behind me because his male 50–59 AG takes off right after my women's 50–59 AG. I wonder how long it will be before he overtakes me. I see him coming up behind me somewhere around the twentieth floor. He is soaked with sweat and breathing hard. I don't know why I'm surprised. It's easy to assume that elites have an easier time of it than the average climber, but I've learned over the years that it's tough for everyone.

I think I've done well, but I can't stick around for the results. I need to head back to Orange County since I work early the next morning. I take a call from Mark in the car on the way home. He is so excited. At the age of fifty-one, he finished in second place *overall* by one second to nineteen-year-old Johnny Ravello. This is the first climb for Johnny Rocket, as we now call him.

Mark then gives me some surprising news. He tells me I finished first in my age group with a time of 17:22. I ask if he's sure; he says yes. It doesn't sink in—I'm sure it must be a mistake. He says he'll pick up my medal at the awards ceremony. I tell him he should probably wait until the next day when the results are official. He says the results *are* official. Poor Mark is trying unsuccessfully to convince me that I finished first in my age group, but I can't believe I've done that well. He picks up my medal that evening.

By the next day, I am ready to accept the fact that I have done very well. I finished fifteenth fastest female overall (elites are ranked separately) out of nearly 250 women finishers. At fifty-four, I am the oldest climber in the top one hundred female finishers. Craig finished in 19:42. Mark zipped up the building in 11:36, second overall out of more than five hundred finishers (not including firefighters) and is still more excited about my finish than his. He's very proud of the progress I've made in my two-and-a-half years of climbing. And so am I!

CHAPTER SEVEN

Unlikely Steps

My experience with organized sports was very limited before I got involved with stair climbing. During my sophomore year in high school, a friend talked me into joining the girl's softball team. We had lots of fun, and I made one big play—catching a high fly ball hit right to me in center field in the last inning that cinched a playoff victory for us in the finals—but it wasn't much as far as a workout.

Having grown up with a pool, I loved to swim and was a member of the swim team my senior year of high school. I was a good swimmer, but not outstandingly fast. Once again, it was fun and I enjoyed the social aspects, but it didn't do much for my body. I weighed 140 pounds when I graduated high school.

The only time I ever worked out as part of an organized program was in 2004. Two people my friend Jana knew wanted to help people get into shape as a ministry. We met on Saturday mornings, listened to a presentation about diet and nutrition, and then exercised for an hour. I cut my carbohydrate intake and portion size, worked out a couple hours a week at the gym (my first and only experience with the gym), and walked almost every day. I weighed 240 pounds going in and lost at least twenty.

The most valuable tool I carried away from this experience was the concept of shopping the perimeter of the grocery store, which was discussed one week. I often thought of this during my weight loss, because that's exactly what I did then and still do now. The only items I buy from the center aisles of the store are dog food and cleaning and paper products. All of the items I live on—meat, fish, fruits, vegetables, milk, yogurt, and bread—are found on the perimeter of the store. That's a great thing to keep in mind when shopping. If it's down one of the aisles, you can live without having it on your plate.

In those Saturday morning workouts, we exercised so hard that I would be sore for days. We worked out on machines and ran "ramps"—we would trot down the ramp next to the gym to an empty riverbed and run back up repeatedly. My legs would be so stiff and hurt so badly that I didn't even want to walk the dogs for days after. I hated the feeling of being sore; it not only kept me from working out, but I didn't even go for walks. "No pain, no gain" doesn't work well for me. I hated those Saturday workouts because I knew I would be miserable for days afterward. As soon as the program ended, I stopped going to the gym. It took me a year or so, but I gained all the weight back. And then some.

CHAPTER EIGHT

Two Steps Forward, Three Steps Back

At the age of twenty-nine, I'm single, living in my mother's house, without a job, and in debt. I've made a complete mess of my life; I need a fresh start. In August 1985, Mark calls and suggests I move to California. I argue that it's too far away. I'd rather move to New York, Washington, D.C., or Baltimore. All of the cities I mention are about a four-hour drive from home. Mark says California is as close as those cities, albeit by air. He says I should drive to California and see what I think. I can always go back home if I don't like it. Once again, I don't remember the exact moment I decide to move, but I figure it's worth a try.

My friend Jeff agrees to drive out with me in my car and fly back by himself. I'm a year older than Jeff—he's the same age as my brother Nick. We've known one another since they were in the first grade. We leave Vinco at 9:00 a.m. the Saturday before Labor Day and pull into Fullerton, California, at 10:00 p.m. Monday night. We make it in sixty-one hours, only stopping Sunday night to sleep in a motel (a dump) in Gallup, New Mexico. Jeff spends a week exploring Southern California with me and then flies back home. I like California and decide I'll give living here a try, so I start looking for a job immediately. I apply at twenty restaurants before being hired at La Vie en Rose in Brea. La Vie is a lovely country French restaurant with an Italian maître d' named Bruno, who hires me. I start there two weeks to the day after I arrive.

I live with Mark rent-free until I can pay my way. He shares a house with three roommates who agree that I can stay on the couch until I find a place to live. I can't afford to buy much food and I'm drinking very little, so I lose forty pounds in the first few months. I swim regularly in the pool at the complex where we live.

Mark attends the Evangelical Free Church in Fullerton pastored by Chuck Swindoll. I had listened to Chuck on the radio even before I moved west and am happy to go to church on Sundays. Chuck is an amazing teacher. I enjoy church and make friends there. After a few months Mark and I get a two-bedroom apartment in Brea, a few blocks from EV Free, as it was called. In 1986, I begin going to a group at church called ACA, for adult children of alcoholics. A pastor had made an announcement about the group one Sunday morning. I have no idea what a support group is; I think I'll go to a meeting where I'll learn facts about growing up in an alcoholic home and information on how to fix the issues I'm dealing with in my life. I picture myself with a note pad getting info on what changes I could make to undo the damage that had been done to me during my childhood.

It would not be quite that simple. Instead, I discover a group where it is safe to share what I went through in my family of origin, and I learn that I'm not alone. Our family dynamic was not unique and growing up as I had created issues that were common in those with similar experiences. It is the beginning of an awakening for me as to how my home life had damaged me. For the first time in my life, I feel like I can be the real me and be understood. In this group I meet Becky Caffery, who would become a lifelong friend. Becky introduces me to a wonderful women's Sunday fellowship group there. Becky encourages me to get baptized, and we are both baptized on the same Sunday in the summer of 1987. It would be more than ten years later, though, at Mariners Church in Irvine, when I finally internalize the fact that God truly does love me.

After about a year, I move to my own place at the beach and begin riding my bike at least three miles a day. As a result I lose another ten pounds or so and am happy with my body.

I decided to turn over a new leaf when I made the cross-country move, and I haven't been in a relationship until meeting Ariana's dad, Jack, at Le Biarritz restaurant in Newport Beach where I now wait tables. He frequents the bar, is cute, friendly, and has a sailboat. I am taking sailing lessons at Orange Coast College, so we have a common interest, and after a few months we start dating. When I become pregnant, Jack says he's not interested in being tied down by fatherhood and gives me a choice between him and the baby. He goes as far as giving me a check to pay for an abortion. Needless to say, we're not on the same page. I am devastated, but I decide to have the baby on my own.

I gained about forty pounds with my pregnancy but I lose it all within a few months of Ariana's birth. I go back to riding my bike two weeks after, with her first in a front pack, and then, when she's a toddler, a child's seat.

The weight creeps back on when we hit the stage where she's too big for the back of my bike and too small to ride very far on her own bike. I slack off on riding, and at work I am promoted to a managerial job, which puts me at a desk for much of the day.

I start drinking too much again, because I'm unhappy with my personal life and now have the added pressure of being a single mom having to support not only myself, but a baby. I hit rock bottom when I'm arrested for DUI driving home from work on New Year's Eve 1990. My mother, who is visiting from Pennsylvania to help me with Ariana, has to take a taxi to the police station at 4:00 a.m. New Year's Day with two-year old Ariana in tow. You can imagine how well that goes over.

The next time we all get together, Mark asks Ariana, "How old are you?"

"Two," she replies.

"How many ears do you have?"

"Two."

"How many eyes do you have?"

"Two."

"What was your mom's blood alcohol?"

The response is the same: two. Mark thinks it's the funniest thing ever. The arrest costs me thousands of dollars in fines and increased insurance costs. I have to go to AA meetings and alcohol counseling, and I lose my license for a short time.

Over the next twenty years, I take off a few pounds, then put more back on. I recall being in the ocean one summer day after my weight surpassed two hundred pounds. When I stand up out of the water, I can feel the fat on my body drop on my frame. I've never had that sensation before, and I think this must be what it feels like to wear a "fat suit." If only it was a fat suit! Then, during a routine physical exam, the nurse comments that I should get a flu shot since I'm not healthy. Not healthy? That stings. I've always considered myself to be a very healthy person since I'm rarely sick with a cold or the flu. She is referring to my blood pressure and my weight, which are both much too high. Her comment makes a deep impression on me. By the time I leave the restaurant business, I am a size eighteen and weigh well over two hundred pounds.

I start seeing a therapist, Margarita, in 1993 for help in dealing with anger issues that are affecting my life at home and at work. She tells me I am suffering from anxiety and depression. Margarita says that a home like ours is what produces a new generation of alcoholics or addicts. She recommends I go to a recovery support group at Mariners in addition to my weekly counseling sessions. I begin participating in meetings there in January 1994, after my typical period of resistance. I'm curious about what kind of church offers such an amazing outreach, so I attend a Sunday service there. I love it, and Mariners becomes my home church. The counseling and recovery meetings help me in nearly every area of my life. My mom dies in her sleep on May 1, 1996, two weeks shy of her sixty-fourth birthday. It was a heart attack—so sudden. I'm in shock and go to counseling twice a week for a few weeks until I come to terms with her death. She didn't take care of herself. She would lose a lot of weight whenever she spent time in California with Ariana and me because she ate healthier and was more active. When she would go back to Pennsylvania, she would slip back into unhealthy eating patterns and gain weight. I know she struggled with emotional issues, but she would never talk about them with any of us. My mom was such a people person; she loved meeting and talking to people. She made wonderful friends in our neighborhood on her visits to California. She always tried to have a positive outlook on life—she didn't want to deal with anything negative.

Shortly after my mom's death, Brennan Manning, author of *Abba's Child* and *The Ragamuffin Gospel,* speaks at Mariners several nights over the course of a week. His messages, his sincerity, and his humble, Christ-like attitude allow me to experience God's presence in a very real way. I finally understand that God loves me personally—and not just because he loves everyone. I have always known there was a God; I just didn't know for the first thirty years of my life what that had to do with me. God was big, powerful, and scary. He was up there or out there, and I was down here with my own problems to deal with. Now, thanks to Brennan Manning, I come to understand that God's love has nothing to do with who I am or how good I am; he loves me because *he* is good and perfect.

My goal as a Christian is to walk through each day as closely aligned to God's will for my life as possible. I fail often, but I take satisfaction in knowing that I'm doing the best I can. That's good enough for him, so it's good enough for me.

CHAPTER NINE

Slimming Steps

Beginning during my Encore years, I used fad diets to drop ten or twenty pounds when I needed to. I did the Scarsdale diet many times, the egg diet, the vegetable soup diet, and numerous others—whatever was in the current issue *Cosmo* or popular at the time. I am very good at dieting and always lose weight. I am also very good at putting it back on. As a result of this "yo-yo" dieting, I burn out my thyroid and have been taking Synthroid daily since 2001. This is one of the reasons, along with genetics, that I think I will never be thin again.

In late 2007 I am still not happy with my life, and I resolve to change that fact. I don't exactly know how to go about it, but I decide to change one thing every month beginning the first of the year until I affect real change in my life. Throughout 2008 I set a small, manageable goal for myself each month to change the way I do something. I do little things, such as talking to someone I have a hard time dealing with, getting up earlier, or going to bed earlier. I set walking goals, Bible reading goals, and so on. One month I'm at a loss for what to do, so I change the way I have my hair cut. I want to do anything and everything I can to change the path my life is on. My April 2008 goal is easy: do a stair climb. In December 2008, I quit smoking for good. I was still smoking when I did my first two climbs, which is unimaginable to me now. Each change I make bolsters my resolve and gets me comfortable with tackling new challenges.

I keep up with the monthly change idea, and in January 2009 I decide to lose ten pounds in the ten weeks before the April AON climb. I enlist the help of my friend Jana, who is in terrific shape. At this point, I carry 209 pounds on my five-foot-four-and-three-quarters-inch frame. Jana comes to my house and weighs me each Monday morning. The agreement is that if I don't lose weight, I'll pay her ten dollars. I am too cheap to not lose weight. Instead of eating my usual two eggs and two pieces of whole grain toast for breakfast, I cut out one piece of bread. Jana wants me to eliminate one egg as well, but I'm convinced that I can't survive on just one egg. She suggests a mid-morning snack of a one hundred-calorie granola bar or a yogurt. I've never been a much of a snacker. I normally eat a large breakfast, a nice lunch, and a large dinner, and then eat something later on. My favorite late evening treat is a few big Snyder's hard pretzels with Monterey Jack or blue cheese.

Jana has me eating pretty much the same stuff I usually eat, but fewer carbs and less fat. No pasta (I typically eat a pasta meal at least two or three times a week), no white rice or potatoes, just the one piece of bread daily, no croutons (Caesar salad is a favorite), low-fat salad dressings, and definitely no pretzels and cheese. I walk at least half an hour a day, usually more; I do stairs and drink more water. She also asks me to give up half & half and drink my daily pot of decaf coffee black: no cream, no sugar, no calories! I've never been able to drink black coffee, but I agree to give it a try. I get used to it quickly. Over the course of ten weeks, I lose a smidge over ten pounds, bringing my weight down to just under two hundred pounds. I'm thrilled! By keeping up this eating plan, I continue to maintain my weight, but I don't step on a scale again for nine more months.

In early 2010 my new church, Newport Church, sponsors a ten-week weight-loss program based on the book *Body & Soul* written by our pastor's wife, Dianne Wilson (or "Di" as she's called). At my first weigh-in for the Body & Soul course in late January, I'm 192.8 pounds. I am surprised and very happy. I was worried that I'd put on weight in the time that had passed, but I have managed to lose almost a pound a month by sticking with the basic changes I'd made a year earlier working with Jana.

The *Body & Soul* book focuses on eating healthy and nourishing your soul at the same time by finding freedom in getting healthy and being fit. The eating plan is modeled after the Lindora diet, focusing on higher protein intake and lower carbs. I follow the plan to the letter, walking or climbing stairs every day, eating the prescribed foods, and drinking plenty of water. I don't weigh myself at home, but weigh in before the meeting on Monday evenings. Each week for ten weeks, I get on the scale thinking I won't be any lighter. I'm delighted each week to lose approximately two pounds. One week I lose slightly less, one week more than three, so by the end of the ten weeks, I weigh almost twenty-two pounds less than when I started. I tell Ariana, now a senior in college, during a phone conversation that I really think I can "keep it up," and for the first time in decades, I think it's possible to get my weight down to a normal, healthy range. I continue to follow the program and weigh 162 pounds by the time Ariana graduates in May. I reach my lowest weight of 138.5 pounds in late September. I try to get to 135, but even eating exactly what I'm supposed to eat and running and climbing, I cannot get below 138.5.

It's tough and requires lots of sacrifice. I have to eat differently from everyone else. Especially when going out to eat with a group of people, it's hard not eating burgers, bread, chips and salsa, fries, and so forth. It takes a lot of willpower, but it works—and that makes all the suffering worthwhile.

Everyone in the office knows I'm following an eating plan, and I'm attuned to what they're eating. There are times when my face literally hurts from hunger. During one of those days, my coworker Cheryl walks into the office carrying a small white pizza box from Laventina's Pizza down the street. I watch her come through the door, and I ask her what's in the box. Without missing a beat, she replies "lettuce" and keeps right on walking to the back office where, out of sight, she eats what I know is a hot, delicious piece of pizza.

Di's husband Jonathan jokingly refers to the Body & Soul program as "Protein Prison." He preaches an unrelated but apropos message on momentum during my weight loss. It is so much easier to keep losing weight when you get a good momentum going. It's way easier to lose ten pounds after losing twenty or thirty than it is to lose five pounds after gaining ten. Every time I lose another ten pounds, I search Di out on the patio at church and bound up to her, yelling, "Ten more!" I get a big smile in return.

Going clothes shopping is fun for the first time in years. I take an article of clothing into the dressing room, try it on, and have to ask the clerk to fetch me a smaller size. I cannot begin to put on paper how good that feels. There are at least two occasions when I let out a "woo hoo!"—once when a size eight dress fits beautifully, and another when I slip comfortably into a size six pair of leggings. My wardrobe before losing weight was composed mainly of black items because black is more flattering. I'm now excited to buy brightly colored clothing that looks good on me. I buy new jeans twice during the weight loss process. I want to feel good and attractive in my clothing, not walk around with baggy pants. I sell those nearly new jeans and my "fat clothes" through a consignment shop and use that money to start a new wardrobe.

I also fit into clothes that I've had for over twenty years. A few are basic enough that I can wear them again. I have "fashion shows" and try things on to show Ariana. Lots of them look ridiculous, especially one pair of Chic jeans from the eighties, but it's great knowing I can fit into clothes I've had since my twenties and thirties. Someone once said, "Nothing tastes as good as thin feels," and as hard as that is to remember day after day, it's so true.

Many people compliment me throughout this process, which means a lot to me and is very encouraging when I struggle with hunger. I stop at my local Starbucks one day after climbing practice (black coffee has few calories), and the cute little barista says, "I want to look like you when I'm your age." She makes my day! My doctor's jaw drops the first time he sees me post-transformation. He says, "You must have lost fifty pounds!" At that point, I'd lost fifty-five. He then asks, with raised eyebrows, how I did it. He was relieved when I told him I did it by eating less and exercising more.

Quite a few people cautiously ask if I'm "okay" when they first see the new me, thinking I lost the weight due to illness. My youngest brother Paul accuses me of being anorexic when he first sees me thin. Another friend who hasn't seen me for years asks if I'm anorexic or bulimic. "Which one is it?" she says. I respond with the truth—I'm eating less and exercising more. It's hurtful to have to defend myself on these occasions, but thankfully, those people are in the minority. One neighbor thinks she's complimenting me, I'm sure, when she tells me I have the body of a twenty year-old and that "the past couple of years have really been good to you."

Really, I think later that day, *time has been good to me?* I hate to break it to her, but time is my enemy. I worked very hard to lose the excess weight and get into great shape. Standing passively by while time did its thing is not what has taken place in my life. Getting up at the crack of dawn and trying to milk the most out of each day to get myself strong and healthy is more like it.

The first time I get a haircut, my hairdresser of over ten years, Tatiana, can't believe the transformation. She is an attractive woman but has struggled with her weight off and on during the time I've known her. She asks me question after question about how I've done it. "How long did it take? What are you eating?" she wants to know. "Aren't you hungry?"

I tell her I've had an egg, toast, two servings of yogurt, two apples, a can of tuna, green beans, and salad so far that day, and I am going home after my haircut to eat chicken, salad, and vegetables for dinner. She tells me what she's eaten that day, which is next to nothing. She is forcing her body to conserve energy by not feeding it. The way I eat and exercise encourages my body to burn calories by providing it with healthy food as fuel regularly throughout the day and keeping it in motion to burn off that fuel.

The first thing I do every morning throughout my weight loss is pop a sublingual B12 tablet under my tongue. There is no scientific evidence that

B12 contributes to weight loss, but B12 can help improve energy levels in those with a B12 deficiency. Feeling more energetic can lead to being more active, which in turn should increase overall fitness. I believe it has helped me.

For the first few years of this plan, I eat one egg, usually soft-boiled or poached, and one piece of dry toast (whole grain) for breakfast every day. The sprouted grain, flourless varieties of bread work best with my body. A popular brand is Ezekiel, but Trader Joe's offers several types as well. Their sprouted rye is my favorite. Now I eat half a cup of egg whites instead of one egg. The whites have about as many calories as one whole egg, no fat, and they sustain me longer. I like to use a couple of tablespoons of salsa or pico de gallo on my egg whites. It adds flavor without adding many calories, and it contains no fat. Every day I eat a mid-morning and mid-afternoon snack of six ounces of homemade fat-free yogurt and a piece of fruit, usually a mandarin orange or an apple.

After spending sixteen to twenty dollars a week on Greek yogurt, I start making my own in mid-2010. Commercially prepared yogurt usually has added sugar, while my homemade is nothing but milk. I make a gallon of yogurt a week from a gallon of nonfat milk, which I strain down to half a gallon of Greek style yogurt or yogurt cheese. The whey that is strained off contains much of the carbohydrates, so Greek yogurt has fewer carbs and a higher percentage of protein than regular yogurt. My homemade yogurt costs about forty cents per six-ounce serving, averaging around four dollars a week.

I love pears, and I eat berries when they're affordable and in season. I eat bananas and carrots sparingly due to their high glycemic index. Foods with a high glycemic index spike one's blood sugar and don't provide long-lasting satisfaction compared with other fruits and vegetables. I do sometimes crave bananas, and when that happens, I assume that perhaps my potassium levels are low, so I indulge my craving. I have a hankering for bananas the week before my first Willis climb, so I eat as many as I want that week.

Lunch most every day is half a grilled chicken breast (four to five ounces), two cups of greens (usually spring mix) and fat-free or low-fat dressing and a cup of vegetables—typically fresh green beans or raw broccoli slaw. I add sliced cucumbers, bell peppers, red onions, some shredded zucchini, sprouts, or scallions to keep it interesting. My friend Jana introduced me to Galeos dressings during the Body & Soul program. They are made locally in Costa Mesa and are low-fat and very flavorful. When eating out, I sometimes use salsa or pico de gallo in place of salad dressing. It adds only a few calories and contains no fat. Soy sauce is terrific, too, with lemon juice or balsamic vinegar and a drizzle of olive oil. I usually just use oil and vinegar with soy sauce now, but occasionally I buy Bolthouse Farms yogurt-based low-fat dressings, also very tasty. My favorite used to be the blue cheese variety, but I like their Caesar dressing, too. I add their ranch dressing to shredded cabbage along with some fat-free yogurt and a little cider vinegar when I crave coleslaw. It's pretty darned good.

I might also have a four- to five-ounce burger patty (no bun!) of 93 to 96 percent lean ground beef, lean ground turkey, or a chicken breast or left-over salmon or turkey. A little barbeque sauce adds fat-free flavor, but does have sugar. A can of albacore tuna or salmon works, too. I can't eat regular canned tuna anymore after eating albacore—I might as well eat cat food. Dinner is spring mix with dressing, a vegetable or two and five or six ounces of lean protein, usually a small piece of steak, chicken breast, or fish. When I eat out, I usually have fish. A baked sweet potato with a big squeeze of fresh lime juice adds carbs but is fat-free. A dollop of fat-free Greek yogurt replaces sour cream or mayonnaise. I add spring mix, arugula, spinach, or blanched riced cauliflower to replace rice when I make stir-fry or curried dishes.

Preparation is the key to success for me. If I do not have my next meal planned out or have fruit and yogurt available, I will eat whatever is at hand, and that can get me into a lot of trouble calorie- and carb-wise. I have to buy and cook enough food to cover my next day's lunch so I'm not tempted to eat something I shouldn't.

I get called for jury duty in fall 2010. I'm worried about how I'll deal with eating during that time. I pack an insulated bag with an ice pack and take all the food I need each day with me. The breaks we take jive with my 10:30 a.m. and 3:30 p.m. snack times. I also take the stairs in the courthouse in the morning, at breaks, and during lunch, thus managing to get hundreds of stairs in each day. I don't gain an ounce during my weeks as a juror.

I eat the same thing day in and day out, with endless variations. I get bored once in awhile, but there's so much variety in my simple eating plan that I seldom eat exactly the same meal twice. That's very important to me. Food has been such an important part of my life both personally and professionally. The one little "cheat" I have always allowed myself— even during the ten weeks of the strict Body & Soul classes—are the food samples at Trader Joe's. I figure that one bite of even butter with whipped cream on top is still only one bite. It never hurts me; on the contrary it helps me feel more "normal" and less deprived. When eating out at restaurants that serve generous portions, I ask for a take-out container and put half of my meal in it as soon as my food is served. My meal now has half the calories, half the fat, and half the carbs—and I have lunch or dinner for the next day.

I can't forget to mention water! I drink so much more water now than ever before. I drink filtered water at home and have a full glass of ice water as soon as I wake up. I then drink at least two more glasses before I leave the house, as well as a cup of decaf coffee. I drink another ten or twelve ounces of water before my morning snack and then as much as I can drink throughout the rest of the day. If I get bored, I add a sprig of fresh mint or a slice of citrus fruit or cucumber.

I was never a big water drinker until I began Body & Soul. It makes a world of difference. The dispensed water where I work is ice cold and really quenches my thirst as well as squelches my appetite. At home I drink water with lots of ice and some cucumber, lemon, or lime and mint, if I have it. If I'm having a particularly "hungry" day where I have nagging hunger for long periods, I drink more cold water. When I want to eat something I shouldn't, I'll tell myself to go get some water instead. I think, *Nah, it won't help—I really need food.* But within minutes of drinking a glass of water, I feel much better. It doesn't always work, but most of the time it does. Gum helps, too—a lot. I chew sugarless gum almost every day at work. It keeps me from thinking that I must have something to eat. If I go to an evening event where I suspect I will be tempted to nibble, I brush my teeth beforehand. There's no food I can think of that is worth me brushing my teeth a second time!

I love soup, but so many are loaded with cream and calories. I experimented and came up with a fast and easy three-ingredient soup recipe: Steam veggies such as cauliflower, broccoli, butternut squash, or carrots. Put the vegetables in a blender with the cooking liquid. You may need to add more water to reach the right consistency. Puree with an immersion blender or traditional blender. Be careful—start off at low speed; the top can blow off when you start to blend if the liquid is too hot. Add Better Than Bouillon chicken or vegetable base (start with half a teaspoon and add more to taste) and a scant teaspoon of powdered nonfat dry milk (optional). Cauliflower soup dressed up with a sprinkle of nutmeg is my favorite. I add a dollop of Greek yogurt and nutmeg to the butternut squash or carrot soup. Zucchini works, too, but add some sliced onion when steaming. Not only is this soup satisfying, it's 99 percent fat-free.

I've also learned to be okay with being hungry. I'm not always comfortable with hunger, but I reached a good place when I was losing all the weight. My hunger was a positive sign that the eating plan was working, and the hunger pangs assured me that I was losing weight. I still struggle with hunger every single day. I thought that once I got to a normal weight,

I would feel differently, but I don't. I'm hungry pretty much all of the time, except when I've just eaten, and I could almost always keep eating. Of course now I rarely ever eat to the point of being full—it's way too uncomfortable. I judge how much I will eat, not by what my stomach tells me, but by the portion I've allowed myself on my plate. I used a kitchen scale to weigh nearly everything I ate when I was on Body & Soul. It made me realize what huge portions I had been eating for all those years.

If I want pizza now, I order one slice. We used to order a whole pizza, and I'd eat half. I don't think we've had a whole pizza in our house since 2010. The first time I allowed myself to have pasta after my weight loss, it was corn pasta. I eat that or brown rice or whole-wheat pasta occasionally, and sometimes soba (buckwheat) noodles (my favorite) rather than pasta made from white flour. I read on the package that a serving was two ounces, and I weighed out one portion. I boiled the water and added the pasta. My reaction was, "Are you kidding me?" What a waste, I thought, to boil water to cook such a small amount of food. When it was done, I added steamed broccoli, chunks of grilled chicken breast, a fourth of a cup of marinara sauce (check the label—basic tomato and basil sauces can be nearly fat-free), a sprinkle of Parmesan cheese, and voilà! I had a large satisfying bowl of pasta. I was discovering how delicious eating healthy can be.

CHAPTER TEN

Climbing Pittsburgh

On Christmas Day 2010 Ariana and I spend the evening with Mark and his family. We talk about stair climbing with one of Mark's sisters-in-law who has done a couple of climbs with us in the past. She's in my age group. As I walk across the room to check out an array of desserts they had prepared (yes, I had a couple of pieces), I overhear her tell Mark that she should start training and do another climb. She says, "I bet I can beat your sister." He shakes his head and says, "No way." She says if she trains hard she can. Mark responds with, "She'll kick your ass." I secretly smile an extremely big smile.

Mark tells me he's going to participate in the American Lung Association Climb in Pittsburgh in March and says I should do it, too. Initially I say no (hard to believe); I have no intentions of flying back east. I've never done a race outside of LA. Later that week I decide to take two weeks off and schedule a visit home to coincide with the climb. I haven't been back to Western Pennsylvania for six years—I am overdue for a visit with friends and family. I'm in good shape, right around my target weight of 140 pounds. I want to fly back, participate in the race, and spend the remainder of the two weeks visiting family and friends. I end up having to go back two weeks before the climb due to my friends' schedule. I worry about completing my training there and what I'll eat. Western Pennsylvania isn't exactly known for healthy cuisine, and I want to enjoy some of those fat- and carb-rich foods from my childhood while I'm there. My sister has opened a pizza shop since I'd been home last. I want to try her pizza, as well as a deep-fried cinnamon roll she makes that I'm anxious to sample. (The pizza was very good and the deep-fried cinnamon roll topped with ice cream was fantastic). I want to enjoy my trip and at the same time not undermine all the hard work I've done to get ready for this climb.

I want to build my stamina. The best way I can think of to do this is to increase the number of stairs in a row that I climb. I have been training on a flight of 250 stairs. There's a big difference between climbing three repetitions of one hundred stairs and climbing three hundred in a row. The greater number of stairs in a row, the higher your heart rate and the more strenuous your breathing becomes since you don't get a break between trips.

I ask security at the tallest nearby building in Costa Mesa if I can use the stairs there. He says no way. I ask at another building in Newport and am turned away there as well. As a climber I always respect private property and never train in a building without permission. As for public buildings or parking garages, I respect the property, am polite and quiet in my comings and goings, and never create any kind of disturbance or commotion. I use common courtesy.

In January I finally find a tall building in Newport Beach where the security guard lets me climb the stairwells. I wear my team West Coast Labels T-shirt when I approach him for permission so he will take me seriously. I consider wearing a couple of my medals but think that might be overkill. He jokes that if he was a good security guard, he wouldn't let me into the stairwell, but he allows local firefighters to use the stairs there for training, so he says it will be okay for me to climb there, too.

This building has 320 steps in one stairwell and 328 in the second. I can take the elevator down, but most of the doorways to the individual floors are locked off for security, so I can only access elevators on certain levels. I climb to the top, take stairs back down to the first open door, exit to the elevator, go back down and repeat. I was asked by security to take the service elevator in a hallway at the opposite end of the building. If I forget to wear my gloves, I have to break after three or four ascents to wash my hands. I wear football receiver gloves to improve my grip on the handrails, but they also prevent me from getting my hands sweaty and dirty from the rails. These stairs are used so infrequently that the railings are coated with dirt and dust, and my hands get filthy. Oh, the obstacles one must overcome to climb!

One day I encounter a young guy trapped in the stairwell around the third or fourth floor. I assume he's a visitor who accidentally locked himself in before he realized that, once you're in the stairwell, you cannot exit without a key card. I rarely run into anyone on the stairs there and I am listening to music, so he startles me. He asks if I have a key to get out as I pass by. I say no and keep going. I call back to him, telling him he can follow me up to an open doorway. He gives me a puzzled look and pulls out his cell phone. I'm sure he thinks I'm strange, but I think he's the strange one for choosing to stand in the stairway and call for help rather than climb up a few floors to get out.

I start with two or three trips up the building the first time and build up to six or more reps by the time I fly home to do the Pittsburgh climb. What a great workout! I also start walking backward and climbing stairs backward. I don't exactly know what that's doing for me, but I figure it can't hurt.

One rainy morning I head over to the building but I really, really do not want to climb. Some days it's awfully hard to get motivated and push myself physically. I know it's going to be painful, and today I just don't think I can do it. I pull out my phone and go to our "Stair Race Training Buds" page on Facebook. There we share stories about climbs, training, injuries, and victories. I post that I'm sitting outside the building in my car, and I don't want to go in. Within seconds fellow climbers from all over the country post messages of encouragement such as "Just do it!" and I muster the courage to work out. The anticipation of the pain of climbing is usually a lot worse than the real thing. Once I get into the stairwell and get going, I'm fine.

Ariana and I are watching TV one evening when they show a shot of the LA skyline. I hit the pause button on the DVR and say, "Look at that!" She asks what she's supposed to look at.

"Look at those tall buildings," I say. "Can you imagine that someone's mother has climbed the two tallest buildings there multiple times? She must be amazing!" Ariana shakes her head and rolls her eyes in response.

Come March, I fly home and stay with friends. For the first week, I cheat on my diet a bit and drink alcohol, which I usually do not do. It's a waste of calories. At one hundred calories, a four-ounce glass of red wine is the best option. And I don't know about you, but I seldom drink just four ounces of wine. In addition, your body cannot store calories ingested in alcohol form, so you must burn those first.

While I'm in Pennsylvania, I run two miles almost every morning, some mornings in the snow. My fingers are freezing even with gloves on; it's twenty-eight-degrees. The coldest temperature I'm used to running in at home is above forty. At least one morning I run part of the way with my hands tucked in my armpits. I drive downtown to a parking garage and run stairwells there. There are eighty stairs total, so I do ten to twelve ascents a couple of times over the course of the week. I like to train to the climb—if a race has a thousand steps, I'll do a minimum of twelve hundred or more at a time in the last few weeks of training.

The afternoon before the race, I make the hour-long drive to Pittsburgh. Mark has recommended the Omni William Penn Hotel downtown where he is staying, so I've reserved a room there. It's beautiful. I ask to switch rooms because the first one is located next to the elevators, which chime when the cars arrive. Even though they shut down at a decent hour, I'm going to bed early and need to know I can get an uninterrupted night's sleep. They give me a room in the farthest corner of the hotel, which is fine with me. The morning of the race, I eat yogurt and a few blueberries (I requested a room with a fridge so I could bring my own food) and head for the Gulf Building where the climb, benefitting the American Lung Association, takes place.

The Gulf Building is only a block or so from the hotel, but I get lost! It has a distinctive roof, which is easy to spot—except when you're at street level beside it. Duh! I end up running several blocks around the area twice before I find the entrance. I'm embarrassed about getting lost, but I get a nice little warm up in the process, which I later think likely added to my performance that day.

At thirty-seven floors, this will be the shortest climb I've ever done. I know I'll have to be fast; on the taller buildings stamina is more important than speed. I don't know how I'll do in a building half the size of U.S. Bank. The lobby area inside the Gulf Building is very small, and there's not much room for climbers to spread out. We all collect in an entryway where we get our bibs, numbered in order of start, and are given instructions. We're supposed to line up according to our bib numbers, and I'm number 184. As usual there are very few elite competitive runners slated to take off first. Most climbers are in teams set up to support a specific recipient or in corporate groups of co-workers, etc. I don't want to have to pass a large number of climbers ("traffic" in climbing lingo), so I sneak in behind number 17, hoping that if they're checking, they'll see just the first two digits of my bib and let me go. No one notices. This is a smaller climb, three hundred plus participants, so the start is casual. It's still chilly outside, but happily this building has an inside start. We enter a very small, dark hall and wait for the word to start.

Each of us takes off in turn. I'm surprised to pass quite a few people on the initial couple of floors. I'd told Mark the night before that I thought I could do the thirty-seven floors in about six minutes or so. That's my goal. The stairs are hard and cold, maybe marble, and the stairwells themselves are narrow and rather dark—it's an old building. I'm able to use the handrails, which I think are brass, quite a bit. As usual, I'm preoccupied with my heavy breathing and burning quads. I am focused and never look up until the twenty-fourth floor. I'm happy to know I'm about two-thirds of the way up. I do not remember crossing the finish line; I don't remember hitting the top of the stairwell. I snap out of it when I step out into the cold air and sunshine at the top. Mark and Rich Burgunder have finished and are walking around on the walkway rimming the roof. I don't know anyone else up there.

My knees are wobbly, so I walk the narrow pathway around the top of the building, take some photos with my phone, and relax a bit. I forgot to wear my watch, but I estimate from calculating the times of the songs I listened to on my iPod that I've done it in about seven minutes. I am happy with that, so I take the elevator downstairs where the climbers are directed to a room with drinks, fruit, and bagels. This is the first climb where I notice they have alcohol: beer. It's not even 9:00 a.m., so I stick with water and decaf. We mill around, chat, and take photos for about an hour while the other climbers finish. Then we move into another room for the awards ceremony, where Mark is announced as the overall winner of the event with a time of 4:43. I'm not surprised.

When they announce the name of the fastest female climber with a time of 6:54, they say my name! I'm flabbergasted! I cannot believe my ears. Both Mark and I receive great first place medals, and we also receive one of four medals given to the four fastest members of the fastest team. Our team that day is made up of a group of mostly Central Cambria High School alumni from Ebensburg, Pennsylvania, where we had attended high school. They chose to name the team "The Pittsburgh Stairlers." Mark is, once again, more excited than I am about my win and gives me high-fives every time I see him throughout the day.

This is an especially sweet victory, being that this race is on my "home turf" in Pennsylvania. This is also a first in tower racing: the first (and perhaps only) time a brother and sister place first overall in the male and female categories. The guys at towerrunning.com dub it "Trahanovsky Day" on their global website. I finish eleventh overall and move into the World Cup Top 50 Female Climbers in the world (*in the world!*) as a result of this climb, and I could not be more ecstatic. All my hard work and sacrifice has paid off. It's a great feeling to achieve first place. I still question whether I could have done it faster, but this time it doesn't matter. Mark has a nice Lucite trophy made for my birthday in May commemorating my first (and so far only) fastest overall female finish. I am now determined to excel in April in my fourth trip up the AON Building back in LA.

Sebastian Wurster is the statistics guy at www.towerrunning.com, the internationally recognized website that tracks every single climber in every one of the hundreds of races that take place each year around the globe. He presented his first official rankings in 2009 and included women in the rankings in 2010 for the first time.

Sebastian was a very bright elementary school student in Germany when, out of boredom, he began keeping track of which student got back to their seat first after their lunch break. When his schoolmates discovered what he was doing, they began racing up the staircase back to the classroom to see who would be first. He developed a system of assigning points to determine rankings. Sebastian would hold quarterly finals and then name a winner at the end of the term. He continued this ranking system throughout his school years until he graduated from high school in 2006. Coincidentally, in 2006 Thomas Dold of Germany won the Empire State Building RunUp in New York City, which made headlines in Europe. Sebastian was shocked to find out that staircase racing, as he calls it, was an organized sport, and he decided to learn everything he could about it. He began tracking all the races and applied his scoring techniques to climbers, assigning each climber points based on their order of finish. Today, towerrunning.com is the most comprehensive source of stair climbing information in the world. If you want to find a climb near you, no matter where you are, visit towerrunning.com.

Once home from my Pittsburgh trip, I have four weeks to prepare for AON 2011. I keep up my usual training routine until early in the week of the race. If race day is Saturday, the Monday prior is the last day I do stairs, and Wednesday morning is the last run for the week. All I do Thursday and Friday is walk the dogs and relax. By Saturday morning, I'm raring to go. This is the case for AON on April 30. I am well rested, well trained, in good shape, fresh off my Pittsburgh victory, and confident about my chances for a medal in my age group. I have a good position at the start and have a good climb. On the way up I swear I will never do another climb; it's too hard, I'm too old, and why did I ever let Mark talk me into this? But I experience this every climb when the going gets tough. As soon as I cross the finish line, all of those thoughts are completely forgotten until about halfway up the next building.

When I get to the top, I spend a few minutes taking photos. After about ten minutes, we are asked to go down to the hospitality area a few floors below to minimize the number of people on the roof. Lisa Zeigel and Karen Geninatti, challengers in my age group, are there, and we compare times. I know Lisa beat me. She's two years younger than I am and is always faster than I am. Karen, who had flown in from Chicago for the climb, says she did it in fewer than thirteen minutes. I'm bummed. I had expected to be second, but now am at least third in my age group. When the final results come in, I finished in 13:31, Karen in 12:57; Lisa, 12:49. I'm the eleventh female overall: number 9 had 13:29; number 10, 13:30. We're separated by one second each. Ugh!

I dropped my sunglasses on the way up, and I am now tortured wondering whether stooping down to pick them up had cost me a place in the top ten. After my initial disappointment wears off, I realize that the three of us "over-fifty" women have finished in the top eleven. The two women who beat me by seconds are both thirty years old, and I was literally on their heels. Both of the faster women in my age group are personal trainers who work every day at staying in fabulous shape. I hadn't set foot in a gym once in my training. I have much to feel good about.

In case you haven't noticed yet, age isn't a big hindrance in vertical races. Climb times are more about overall fitness than age. Many of the world's top climbers are over fifty; most are over thirty. Twenty-two of the current top one hundred climbers in the U.S. (top fifty males and top fifty females) are under thirty; fifteen are fifty and older. Two of those are men in their sixties, and there's even one seventy-year-old! Mark ranks twenty-fifth on towerunning.com's top thirty male climbers in the world 2009–2014. He is one of seven American climbers on the list. Towerrunning.com does not list an athlete's age, so I don't know how many are over forty or over fifty on that list.

George Burnham of Phoenix, fondly called "Cowboy George" by his step-sibs due to the fact that he often wears a cowboy hat while climbing, completed his one hundredth stair climb in August of 2014 at the age of seventy-one. George, a retired carpenter and electrician from Phoenix, competes nearly every weekend, often doing one climb on Saturday and flying to another city to do a Sunday climb. George has accomplished this despite having suffered with asthma for most of his life and undergoing bypass surgery in 2013.

Eighty-year-old Wayne Hunkins of Beverly Hills began stair climbing when he passed a parking structure during walks. He started walking regularly to keep limber and thought that throwing in a few stairs might be of benefit, so he added stairs in a nearby parking garage to his routine. While taking a tour of the Empire State Building on a trip to New York City, he was surprised to learn that there was a competitive climb held there each February. It took some doing and a sizeable cash contribution, but Wayne participated in the Empire State Building Run-Up in 2013. His time was 28:30 for the eighty-six floors (their website incorrectly states that it's 86 *flights*), and he made international news as a result.

Even though they're speedy, these climbers often win age group medals just for showing up and making it to the top.

They could use some more competition.

CHAPTER ELEVEN

A Step Back

After the 2011 AON Climb, I reassess my stair-climbing goals. I had finished third behind two personal trainers, both who are younger than I am. I'm in good shape, but know I can be more fit. I work hard to keep off excess weight, but I cheat on my healthy diet, too. I've been eating dessert almost every day; I have an issue with sweets—I'm a sugar-aholic. If I eat one piece of candy after lunch, I'll eat ten. I know I can be a better climber if I better control my eating.

I tell Ariana if I'm going to work this hard at being a good stair climber, I want to give it all I have and try to really excel. I've been eleventh in female finishers at least twice—I am ready to move into the top ten on the bigger climbs. I begin running five or six mornings a week, between a mile and a half and two miles. I practice on the stairs three times a week. I climb between 750 and a thousand stairs twice a week and way more on Mondays, between a thousand and two thousand. I ride my bike regularly plus volunteer at the local vet's office walking dogs half an hour five mornings a week. I also walk two miles on Mondays with my two little dogs and occasionally during the week. When I train at the seventeen-story building, I start out intending to do five or six trips and when I "finish," I add another trip just to see how much more I can sweat. I'm addicted; I'm obsessed with pushing my limits.

I eat sweets occasionally and even have a glass of wine or a drink now and then, but the extra exercise wipes out the evidence. I buy a size-eight bikini, which I wear proudly to the beach. I'm still far from having a "six-pack," but I am in the best shape of my life.

I usually run first thing in the morning. I set my alarm each morning for 6:15, get dressed, and hit the pavement immediately. I like this time of day best for running because there are fewer people out and about, it's cooler

(I get overheated quickly when I run), and it's gorgeous at daybreak. I often run to the top of a nearby hill just in time to see the sun peek out over the foothills and light up the harbor. It's still my favorite path for walking or running. The beachfront boardwalk is excellent as well. On clear mornings I can see south for miles and miles, with the lifeguard towers silhouetted against the crashing surf and brightening eastern sky. I also don't have time to talk myself out of running if I do it first thing in the morning. It's the hardest thing I do all day, and it's over before 7:00 a.m. I also sleep so much better when I begin my day with a run.

In late July I notice a funny feeling in my left knee when I run. It feels like there's something in it—a bump or something that makes it ride funny in the socket. After a few days I decide to take a break for a week and see if it improves. I give it a week and try running again, but half a mile from home, I can feel "it" in there again, so I lay off for another week or so. It's uncomfortable, but it's not painful and only bothers me when I run.

I have been trying to meet up with a woman interested in stair climbing since January, and I am finally able to meet her on August 17. I haven't been doing many stairs since my knee has acted up, but figure it'll be fine. We meet at one of my training areas and start up the first flight after I explain that my knee has been bothering me. I tell her about doing "double steps," and she asks what I mean. I take two steps with my left leg to demonstrate. When my foot hits the step, it feels as though my knee explodes. I yell out in pain and "hear" my knee pop. I'm not sure if it's audible to anyone else, but it hurts my head, the sound is so loud. I don't want to flake on her since it's taken so long for us to meet up, so I continue to walk up the steps and do about five or six hundred more stairs. I'm in excruciating pain by the time I get home, and by the next morning, it's even worse. I can barely bend my leg to get into the car to go to work. Once at my desk, I have to extend my knee fully and prop it up on a box under my desk. As long as it's elevated and immobile, I'm fine. Craig asks me to go with him to an appointment, and I'm back in excruciating pain. Each movement of the car brings about stabbing pain in my knee. It's as if someone is trying to saw my leg off from inside my knee joint.

At home I search the cupboards for ibuprofen since I rarely take pain medication. I take what I find and spend the evening on the couch, first trying heat, then cold, to alleviate the pain. I can barely walk my dogs; I have to take very deliberate steps. It takes great effort to step up over the curb with my left leg. Ariana says I've gone "from mom to grandma" overnight.

It takes a few days, but I get in to see my doctor for a referral to an orthopedist. He can tell nothing from X-rays, so he sends me for an MRI.

The MRI shows a slight tear in the meniscus and some thinning of the cartilage, neither of which would cause the excruciating pain I'm suffering. I'm certain I tore the meniscus back in 2004 when I was working out with the couple from church. We were doing lunges when my left foot rolled to the outside and caused extreme pain in my left knee that lasted for months. It eventually faded, so I assumed I had strained or pulled something that had healed itself. Now my ortho refers me to physical therapy, since I don't want to undergo surgery for the meniscal tear. I'm certain that's not what's causing my pain. The U.S. Bank Climb is five weeks away. I'm still set on participating in the race and don't want anything to stand in my way, but I can't even walk without limping.

It is in physical therapy where I finally learn what had happened. Everyone kept asking me what I did to my knee, and I would say, "I don't know; I didn't 'do' anything." It wasn't like I had twisted or hurt it in any one incident. My physical therapist, Rich, tells me that my left hip is out of alignment, which causes my thigh bone to strike the knee joint at an improper angle. All the training I had been doing was causing my knee joint to be pounded from an unnatural angle. I never stretched—I didn't think I had to—and this caused my IT band (a tendon that runs from the hip to the knee on the outside of the thigh) to tighten up to the extent that it was pulling my knee cap off to the left, further causing a misalignment in my knee joint.

Rich prescribes a knee brace along with stretching and strengthening exercises. For six weeks beginning September 9, I exercise two or three mornings a week at the PT facility and every other morning at home until I'm once again able to walk without a limp. At the end of the PT sessions in December, I continue my therapy at home. I stretch first thing every morning and do strengthening exercises five mornings a week. I begin running again a little bit at a time, incorporating running short stretches into my walks with the dogs, until I run a solid one and a half miles on Thanksgiving morning 2011. I can't believe I can run on my leg. At the start of PT when I could barely walk, it seemed impossible; my knee was so fragile.

I do the U.S. Bank Climb, but not competitively. I had already signed up for it (I was committed to the fund-raising), so I go ahead and participate. More than one of my friends asks me why I would climb with an injury—why risk hurting myself more? I talk to my PT, who doesn't see any reason I shouldn't take on the building. I need to do this climb for my emotional well-being. Being off my feet for nearly two months has been very stressful. I was extremely depressed in August and September, wondering if I would be able to run or climb again. I sat on the couch most evenings eating cookies and feeling sorry for myself. If I don't run, I have to watch every morsel of food that goes into my mouth, or I'll gain weight. My body is very fuel-efficient. I have to stay active in order to be able to enjoy any extra food at all. The idea that I might never be able to run again or participate in the sport I had grown to love so much was overwhelming.

I really enjoy this climb and have more fun than during any of my previous climbs. There's no pressure to be fast. I wear my knee brace and climb at a steady pace. I still do double steps with my good leg and am very deliberate about foot placement; I navigate each segment of steps carefully so as not to aggravate my left knee. I cheer the other climbers, even tell a few people along the way about my weight loss, and get my first cardio workout in over a month. It's exhilarating, and I manage to do it in 22:47, faster than the first two times I climbed with two good legs!

After the climb I learn that Lisa Zeigel had recovered from a very similar injury earlier in the year. The camaraderie of the athletes at U.S. Bank is so good for my spirit. Doing this climb and mingling with my teammates gives me hope that I will overcome this injury and continue to pursue the crazy sport of competitive stair climbing.

CHAPTER TWELVE

Step-by-Step

On December 3, 2011, I participate in the CFF Climb of Your Life event in LA, which benefits the Cystic Fibrosis Foundation. There are 230 climbers taking part in this second annual event. Runners climb forty-nine stories (1,285 stairs) in a fifty-one-story building downtown at the corner of Wilshire and Figueroa.

I had set my alarm (two of them, actually) for 6:10 a.m. I awake at 5:40 with a nervous stomach and am not happy to be up so early. After trying to doze off again for a few minutes, I get out of bed and do my stretching and strengthening routine, which despite my best efforts to go faster, still takes me about forty minutes. I then walk the dogs about a mile and a half to loosen up a bit. I eat my usual breakfast of a soft-boiled egg and piece of dry whole grain toast, and then get dressed. I put on my most lightweight leggings and my West Coast Labels/ X-Gym team shirt. Mark is the founder and captain of our West Coast Labels team. He offered to put the logo on my shirt after my third or fourth climb. The jersey makes me a member of the fastest stair-climbing team on earth. I wear running socks and the most lightweight running shoes I own. They don't provide enough support for regular running but are fine for stair climbing. I also grab my gloves, which improve my grip on the rails.

During my first couple of climbs, I was behind so many climbers that I could barely stand to touch the sweaty handrails. Using the handrails can give a climber several seconds' advantage, probably more. Some stairwells have railings on both sides, and climbers can pull themselves up with both arms. We call that "double railing it." Others do not, or the stairway is too wide, with the rails too far apart to reach. Some climbers use a "hand over hand" technique with only one rail to maximize their efforts.

Craig is doing the climb with me today and picks me up at 8:15 a.m. for the drive to LA, and we arrive at 9:15. The first wave of climbers (experienced competitive or "elite" climbers) are due to take off at 9:45. We are preregistered and go directly to check in after parking the car. Most events provide free or reduced-cost parking, and this one is free.

Upon arrival we meet many of our stair climbing "family" members. Getting together at the race is like old home week. After some quick hellos and hugs, Craig and I proceed on to get our bib numbers, which we pin to our jerseys, and then the timing chip which attaches with a zip tie to our shoes through the laces. I also owe a balance on my shortfall for fund-raising. Most climbs require a minimum of $100 to $150 to participate, which goes to the charity sponsoring the event. I used the CFF tool to fund-raise on Facebook and raised $75.00, so I supply a credit card to pay the difference.

When a climber does multiple climbs over the course of a year, it's tough to ask people over and over to contribute money. Most competitive climbers end up paying all the registration fees and fund-raising themselves. Many climbs offer a discount if climbers register far enough ahead. Now that I do six or more events a year, I usually fund-raise on Facebook for just one climb. Competitive climbing is an expensive sport especially if you have to pay airfare, hotel, and meals for an out of town event.

At this point, my hands are shaking so badly that I can barely get the little plastic zip tie onto my shoelace. I have never been this nervous before a climb, and this is my eleventh climb. Mark still gets nervous and sometimes eats Tums to help settle his pre-race butterflies. I have a lot riding on this climb. It'll be my first all-out effort following my knee injury, and I don't know what I'll do if I blow out my knee or otherwise injure it on this climb. I also know that I've only been climbing stairs for a few weeks in preparation. I wish I'd had another several weeks—or ideally a month—to get in more workouts and trim off a few more pounds (I'm almost ten pounds heavier than when I climbed last year). Thankfully my time to worry is short, since there's just enough left to hit the restroom and go outside for a prerace pep talk and a few ground rules.

I hate outdoor starts in cold weather. In the past I have been so cold and nervous that I shake uncontrollably in the car on the way to the race. Ariana drove me to Los Angeles for a climb once, and I made her turn the heat up so high that she had to take off her T-shirt and drive wearing just a sports bra because I was so cold I couldn't stop shaking; I ended up getting a terrible headache. She still brings that up once in awhile, and not in a good way. I was shaking so badly at a spring climb in San Diego with an outdoor start that my lips were quivering and I could barely speak. Mercifully it's not that cold today.

The rule most important to competitive climbers is to stay to the outside if you're a slow climber to allow faster climbers to pass on the inside rail. Slower climbers are encouraged to move away from the inside rail to the wall to allow ease in passing. Since this is a new climb with a smaller number of participants, the start is casual. We all walk around to the other side of the building to access the stairwell. I'm only about eight from the front, standing behind a chubby little woman wearing a yellow T-shirt with some slogan on it that matches other members of one of the teams climbing today. I want to just push in front of her in line so I don't lose precious seconds passing her inside the stairwell, but I obviously can't do that. Mark, PJ, and the very competitive top runners have already gotten the first several spots in line. After they start up the stairs at fifteen-second intervals, I put my arm around yellow T-shirt woman and ask if she's climbing competitively. She's says no, so I ask if she minds me jumping in front of her, and she says okay.

I'm very relieved and soon find myself right behind Lisa Ziegel, up next to take off. I'm glad she's ahead of me. It's very stressful to have a fast climber right behind you because it can throw off your pace, make you climb too fast at the start, and burn out quickly. I had also asked Craig to be sure not to take off right behind me for the same reason. I give Lisa a pat as she takes off. Jeannie grabs my shoulders in encouragement. I never asked her how she got around yellow T-shirt woman. They told me I'd be taking off at 9:57:15. I watch the large digital display hit 15 and take off over the timing mat. I am always careful to hit the mat. At the Gulf Building climb in Pittsburgh in March, climber Rich Burgunder took such a long stride when he took off that his timing chip did not register and he missed out on a medal by the time they found his time through the computer. They do have a back-up timing system, but it takes time to research in case of a problem.

Back at the CFF climb, by the time I get to the tenth floor, my quads start to tighten up. I don't look at the floor numbers for as long as I possibly can—the longer I can keep from looking at the numbers, the faster the climb seems to go—but I know the first water station is on the tenth floor and I notice the volunteers there. Now I spot Jeannie, also in my age group, behind me, and I am stressing big time. She's coming on fast and gets to within eight or ten stairs of catching me. I don't like it one bit. She beat me the first several races we did together, and I finally beat her for the first time in September 2010 at U.S. Bank. She hasn't competed for the past several climbs and had instead focused on running 5ks, at which she excels, so I was extremely worried that she would pass me.

By the time I hit floor fifteen, my quads are on fire and I'm struggling, even though this should be a breeze. I yell, "Shit, shit," and Jeannie says,

"What's wrong?" I say, "This is hard, too hard." I don't know if she replies; I have my earbuds in and the volume cranked up so I can't hear myself breathe or groan. I pass more water stations, and then see someone above the stairway to my right taking photos. All I see are flashes, and then I feel as though they're behind me. Stan Schwarz passes me in there somewhere along with a guy I don't know wearing a red U.S.C. T-shirt. They're the only climbers who pass me on my way up—just the way I like it. I try not to look up, but I finally see the sign on floor forty-four. At some point, Jeannie begins to fade and drops back. I'm in too much pain to care much; I'm giving it all I have. I had forgotten that this building had lots of flights with an uneven number (nine) of stairs. That throws me off a bit since I'm taking two at a time.

Now my lips are parched, my throat is getting sore from breathing so hard, and my legs are screaming for me to stop. I start thinking about each person who has donated to my fund-raising, and then I visualize crossing the mat at the top. I vaguely remember the top from the year before, and I just keep picturing myself getting up there and taking the elevator back down. I hear cheering from above as people cross the finish line, so I know I'm getting close and try to push faster, but I feel like my legs are made of lead and I can't speed up at all. As I hit what I thought was the last turn, I see there are still more stairs ahead. In my training climbs, I always try to speed up on the last segment of stairs, knowing this is it. I do my best to finish hard. When I finally reach the top, I'm gasping for breath, along with everyone else up there. I grab a little Dixie cup of water and drink the whole thing in one gulp. I see a stack of bags of what look like cement, so I stagger over and sit down on one, still struggling to catch my breath.

My daughter had served as a volunteer the year before. Mark gave her a video camera with which to shoot climbers coming across the finish line. She said she quit after about a dozen, because she'd ask them how it was and everyone said, "Terrible," "Awful," "Horrible," and so on. These are my exact sentiments today! I looked at my sports watch before I plopped down, and it read 10:08, so I know I'm right around eleven minutes. I had done 10:38 in 2010 and was hoping to be close to that time. Mark finished today in a little over seven minutes (7:07). Lisa and Jeff are there; Lisa had done it in 9:38. Soon Jeannie (12:14) and Craig (12:38) come up.

After about five minutes, a bunch of us take the elevator down, coughing and hacking all the way. Someone, probably Jeff, jokes that we sound more like a bunch of chain smokers than elite athletes. PJ and Jeff donned paper "surgical" masks for this climb. PJ says that wearing them immediately after the race helps cut down on the particulates you inhale and helps minimize the cough. PJ wore his for at least part of the trip up, but Jeff put his on after. I may give it a try some climb. I'd have paid cash money for some lip balm on my way up, so the mask couldn't hurt.

The next day I still have the "croupy" cough and a minimally sore throat. I had a busy day; if I'd had time to sip some hot tea with lemon, I'm sure the sore throat would be gone by now. It will be tomorrow. The cough is almost gone. I coughed up some mucus earlier today, which helps a lot. As unpleasant as it sounds, it's very common.

After taking the elevator back to the lobby, we join up with climbers as they come down to the courtyard outside the building to enjoy food and beverages provided by sponsors. I have some water, a yummy caffeine-free hibiscus tea sample, and a banana provided by Albertson's grocery store. They have sandwiches, bagels, and adult beverages, but I'm never very hungry immediately after a race and I know that a bunch of us are going out to lunch, so I don't eat anything else. The results are posted quickly. I am disappointed to see that I'd finished in 11:51, 1:13 slower than the year before. At that point, I think I'm twenty-first overall, but as more climbers finish, I move down to thirty-sixth overall, eleventh overall female (again). I'm happy to have medaled in my age group, though: Lisa is first, I'm second, and Jeannie is third. Mark (age fifty-two) finishes third overall behind Eric Leninger at 6:20 (age twenty-eight) and Jesse Berg (age thirty-nine) who finishes in 6:29, despite being as sick as a dog. Mark beat PJ by one second. Top females are Kourtney Dexter, age thirty-one, with 7:16 and Veronica Stocker, age forty-two, with 8:05. Lisa takes third overall female.

This race is of value to me on several levels. First, it's fun mingling with the other climbers. I remember the first time I met climber Nelson Quong at the AON climb in 2011. Nelson was telling a story about going to his car after work to get a change of clothes so he could "do stairs" on his way home. He was speaking my language! My friend and coworker, Stacy, has been climbing stairs with me since the beginning. She hasn't engaged in any of the competitions (yet!); she just likes the benefits of the workout. We'll ask one another if we're "doing stairs" after work. It was so funny to hear someone else use our lingo.

All the regular climbers are so enthusiastic about the sport—getting together is energizing. Everyone, of course, shares stories about their latest climbs, injuries, other sports they compete in (many are also runners and cyclists) and lots of training stories—the torturous regimens we all put ourselves through to perform better in the stairwells. Second, I can see the areas I need to work on to do better on my next climb. I was in better shape when I did the September U.S. Bank Climb than I was for CFF because my "downtime" hadn't affected my conditioning in the five weeks prior to the U.S. Bank Climb as much as it did between then and the CFF Climb. I didn't run once from August 17 until Thanksgiving morning, and I only resumed stair climbing practice after Halloween. It took a toll on me on this climb. I could feel the difference, not only from the weight gain, which cost me at CFF, but also from the terrible tension in my legs. I knew going in that this would be a tough climb for me because I had been having a hard time in practice.

Some of the big climbs sponsor "practice climbs." They'll open up the building or another high-rise to climbers so they can make a practice trip (or trips) to get used to the stairwell or the number of steps. I had not traveled to LA to a practice before this climb, but since then I've done several practice climbs in the AON Building and the Price Waterhouse Coopers Building where the CFF Climb is held. It would have helped a lot in this race. I had forgotten about the stairwells having an uneven number of steps. It helps to know whether the stairwells turn to the left or right, or both—and some switch directions at least for some length of the race at some point. Some climbs have little hallways where you have to sprint to the next staircase. At one AON climb, I "zigged" to the left but had to "zag" right into the correct hallway when I realized I had made a mistake. If a second or two had made a difference in getting a medal for that race, I'd have been ticked. The practices help climbers to be better prepared. Some races have all metal stairs, while others have a mix of cement and metal. Some climbers argue that metal is better; they think you get a bit of a spring from them, while solid stairs are "slower." Each building has its own little nuances that make that particular climb unique.

During one practice at the PWC Building where the CF Climb is held, I was startled when something touched my shoulder. I looked up to see a measuring tape dangling from the floor above and instantly knew Stan Schwarz was on the other end. Stan measures the rise (height) and run (depth) and counts the steps in all the buildings he climbs, as well as "mapping" them. His website, www.1134.org, provides all the twists and turns one can expect to find in the stairwell, as well as the number of steps in each flight of all of those stairways. Stan also calculates how many times up a building equals a vertical mile. In 2014 the race organizers added a "Vertical Mile Club" category at the San Diego Towerthon competition, thanks to Stan.

Familiarity with the buildings helps build confidence and ease prerace jitters. Keeping track of one's times in practice is also useful in training on the tall buildings. It gives the climber an idea of how he or she compares to other climbers and helps with goal setting for race day. As one of my teammates said years ago, "The only way to be a better stair climber is to climb more stairs."

It was at the 2013 CF Climb that I first encountered a teammate climbing without a timing chip. He told me to go ahead and pass; he wasn't doing it for time.

I didn't know what he meant, so I asked him afterward. He explained that he couldn't afford the fees, so he just did it for "fun." At the 2014 U.S. Bank Climb, I ran into a teammate getting ready to go up who was wearing someone else's bib (minus the timing strip) so he could do the climb without paying. Other climbers call this "scabbing." He had maxed out his stair climbing budget for the year and couldn't afford to pay the associated costs. Guys like these love the sport so much they climb even when it doesn't count.

Some climbs are beginning to lower fund-raising minimums for competitive climbers so they can afford to do more races. Competitive climbers are important to organizers because they're the ones who spread the word throughout the stair climbing community and help the climbs grow into national or international events. The fees go to charity, so the money serves a dual purpose. (A portion of the proceeds of each of copy of *See Jane Climb* sold will go to a West Coast Labels/X-Gym scholarship fund to help support climbers like these). The fees go to charity, so the money serves a dual purpose.

CHAPTER THIRTEEN

Thousands and Thousands of Stairs

In January 2012 my friend Kathleen from church invites me to do yoga with a small group of ladies at the clubhouse where she lives. The *idea* of yoga had been appealing to me; actually *doing* it is an entirely different thing. I attend one Monday shortly after I'm invited, and I like it. There are only a few women, all over fifty, and it's very casual. It's also only a half-mile from my house, which is convenient. We exercise to a DVD that focuses mainly on stretching. Ariana comes with me once and dubs it "old lady yoga." It continues to challenge me, so old lady yoga is fine by me.

Yoga helps me remain limber, and helps with my running and climbing. In turn, my climbing and running make my yoga better. I notice during yoga the Monday following a big climb how clear and effortless my breathing is. Breathing heavily during climbs really opens up my lungs, and makes yoga easier. Yoga also has helped strengthen my core. My abs are much more toned since beginning the class.

In April I travel to Europe to spend two weeks with Ariana who is getting her master's degree in Scotland. We fly to Paris for three days and then take the train to London for three days. While trotting after trains and through airports, dragging my bags up and over stairs in the Paris metro, I'm thankful to be in great shape. We climb the Eiffel Tower, the Arche d' Triomphe, Notre Dame Cathedral, and the steps of the Sacré-Coeur all in one day. We walk over eleven miles two of the three days we're in Paris and nine and ten miles a day in London. All the time I spent training for climbs has really come in handy. I joke with Ariana that I thought I was training for stair climbs, but I'd really been training for my trip to Europe. I cannot imagine what my time abroad would have been like without all of my stair training. I do know it would not have been nearly as much fun.

Later that year, Mark designates the second Wednesday of each January as "National Take the Stairs Day." January 9, 2013, is the first "official" National Take the Stairs Day. All those who participate in competitive climbing promote taking the stairs over elevators *every* day, as part of a healthy, active lifestyle, but NTTSD is one day when we make an effort get the message out to as many people as possible. Wednesday is a regular practice day for me; I usually do a thousand stairs after work. I'm not sure how many stairs to do to make this day special. I decide to use the date, 1/9/13, so I do 1,913 stairs after work.

The Sunday before my fifty-seventh birthday that year, a friend at church asks me what I'm doing to celebrate. I tell her I don't have plans; I'm not doing anything special. My birthday falls on a workday, so Ariana and I will probably just go out and have a bite to eat somewhere afterward. I tell my friend that this birthday is kind of an "eh" birthday. Not a "zero" birthday, or an "ends in five" birthday . . . even fifty-six was memorable because I was born in 1956, but fifty-seven is, well, "eh."

Working around the house later that afternoon, I start to think about what I'll do after work on my birthday. What had I done last year? I can't remember. I think that it would be nice to do something to make the day memorable in the years to come. A voice in my head says, "Do 5,700 stairs, a hundred for each year you've been alive." I immediately think, *No way! There's no way I'm doing 5,700 stairs; I work eight hours Wednesday, so there's not enough time even if I wanted to.*

I decide instead to do 5,700 for the week. That's a reasonable goal. I think, *Well that's settled*, but I can't get the idea of doing a hundred for every year out of my mind. It nags at me throughout the day. I argue back and forth in my head for much of the afternoon. The most stairs I've ever done in one day was under three thousand in April at AON when I did a second trip up the building "for fun" with Stan and Lisa. I've done more than two thousand many times. I know I am capable of doing 5,700 stairs in a day, but I don't know how long it will take and I don't have a lot of free time. To climb that many stairs, I'd have to do them on one of my days off. Spreading 5,700 over a week is a reasonable, if wimpy, goal.

I'm scheduled to do a Towerthon in San Diego on June 22. I'll be climbing a twenty-five-story building for two hours. I didn't do the Towerthon last year; I had to work, so this will be my first stair-climbing marathon. Doing 5,700 stairs in one day will be a good warm up for the multi-climb exactly one month away. I want to push myself.

Around six o'clock that night, I finally give in to the idea and tell Ariana, "I have to do 5,700 stairs for my birthday." Nothing much I do surprises her, so her response is a simple "Okay."

I post my idea on our Facebook training page that evening and get a lot of supportive feedback. Most everyone agrees it's a lofty but reasonable goal. A couple of people warn me not to overdo it, to "take it easy." We'll see.

Monday I climb my seventeen-story training building's 328 steps five times for a total of 1,640 stairs. My friend Michele and I do a Monday three-mile pier-to-pier walk later in the day. Tuesday I run a mile and three-quarters first thing in the morning, but I have a full day at work and go out that evening. The run is all the exercise I get that day.

I plan on getting up around 5:30 a.m. Wednesday in order to start climbing by 6:00. I hope to do at least 2,500 stairs before 8:00 a.m., when I'll need to get ready for work. I wake around 4:00 a.m. and try to go back to sleep but can't, so I get out of bed twenty minutes later. I stretch and get to the stairway before 5:30. I plan to climb a nearby five-story parking garage (with a hundred stairs) fifty-seven times. It will be nice and easy to keep track of the numbers that way. I can do 250 stairs each time up if I climb inside the building, but I would have to walk down each time (there is no elevator access inside the building), and I am worried it will be too hard on my left knee, especially given the number of times I'll be climbing the building. The interior stairwell doors are locked on each floor because it's a private, secure building and only employees can access the elevators from the stairwell, which means I must walk back down the entire stairwell after each ascent. I've brought along a large insulated cup of ice water, a towel to wipe away sweat, my iPod, and a small pad of paper and a pen to keep track of how many trips I make. I wear my gloves and a longline sports bra with a tank top over it, Capri yoga pants, and my climbing shoes. I start just after 5:30 a.m. The first several trips are the hardest, as they always are. Once I warm up, it gets easier on my legs, but then my heart rate increases and my breathing becomes more rapid. I eventually fall into a nice rhythm; I'm not in a huge hurry.

After the first thousand stairs, I stop and do a quick series of stretches— hamstring, calf, and quads, thirty seconds each per leg. It's going by faster than I had expected. At 1,500 I've climbed higher than the Los Angeles AON Building. Two hundred more and I've climbed a virtual U.S. Bank. I hit two thousand and stop at the top in the open air to stretch again. Being so early in the morning, the light wind feels wonderful. It's lovely and cool. During the elevator rides down, I post my progress on Facebook via my iPhone and get encouraging messages from other climbers. I have plenty of time to think while climbing and keep track of all the numbers; 2,900 and I've climbed AON twice, two times up U.S. Bank as I hit 3,200. By this time I've taken off my tank top to stay cooler.

Of all mornings, they're doing maintenance on the garage. It doesn't interfere with the first part of the climb, but after about an hour, one worker on the third floor moves very close to the stairwell on his lift and starts painting. I have ample room to maneuver between him and the railing, but the fumes are irritating, especially because I'm breathing so heavily. After thirty-five trips, I stretch and decide to move inside.

Now I'm amped up. I'm getting more and more energized with each repetition. Once inside, doing 250 at a time, I begin sweating like crazy. There are no cool ocean breezes in this stairwell. I switch from rock and roll to worship music. I need all the encouragement I can get! Even with walking back down, the numbers add up quickly. Soon I've completed a thousand stairs and head back outside.

My car is parked on the top floor, so I decide to do a hundred more up to the car before heading home to shower. That makes 4,600. It's almost 7:45 a.m., and I want to stop at Starbucks for a decaf on the way home. As I walk up, I realize that 4,800 would be the equivalent of three times up the U.S. Bank building, so I do two extras, some quick stretches, and then head for home. It had taken me two hours and twenty minutes to complete 4,800 stairs.

After work my coworker Stacy, Ariana, and I change clothes and head up to the parking garage. I stretch and do two trips up by myself. I am very happy to have my two stair climbing training buddies complete the last seven hundred stairs with me. I am elated to have reached my goal and, even better, I finish in plenty of time to go home, change again, and head out to enjoy a terrific birthday dinner. I later calculate that I burned about 1,710 calories on the stairs, which covered *most* of what I ate that day—with the exception of a big piece of birthday cake: chocolate mousse raspberry cheesecake from the Cheesecake Factory.

I climb a little over a thousand more stairs that Friday and 1,640 on Saturday for a total of 10,004 stairs for the week. At first 5,700 seemed like such a high number, but as they say, each journey begins with a single step and all those steps (albeit doubles!) added up quickly. I vow never again to do fewer than a thousand stairs during practice. I have gotten lazy and was doing only six or seven hundred after work. I also decide to switch my focus from running back to stairs. I had been running a lot to improve my climbing, and in so doing, my focus had shifted away from stair climbing. I had forgotten how exhilarating it felt to "reach new heights" in climbing, and I realize that my first love will always be stair climbing.

I am so invigorated and so satisfied with what I accomplished that I've done a hundred stairs for each year on my birthday ever since, and I plan on making this an annual birthday tradition for as long as I'm able.

CHAPTER FOURTEEN

Two Hours of Steps

June 22, 2013, is the date of the Towerthon benefitting Father Joe's Villages in San Diego. For this event, the challenge is to repeatedly climb a twenty-five-story building for two hours to see how many trips up a climber can complete within that time frame. Other climbs across the country sponsor similar events; many are called "Power Hour" climbs. Today's climb also offers the option of doing an "elite sprint" early in the morning for anyone who wants to participate. Last year I only did the sprint. I got up before dawn to drive ninety-five miles to San Diego, climbed for less than five minutes, and drove ninety-five miles back home to go to work. This year I take a vacation day and enter to compete in both races. Half the fun of participating is mingling with my teammates. Today I'll have plenty of time to do that.

Friday night I drive to Carlsbad, more than halfway between my home and San Diego, and spend the night with friends there. I wake just before 6:00 a.m. and put on my gear. I eat as little as possible the morning of a climb, so I've brought along about six ounces of my homemade yogurt to eat in the car on the thirty-minute drive to San Diego. The event will take place downtown at San Diego's Civic Center. For some reason the organizers have decided to have us climb only twenty-four floors this year. This interferes with the times of those who climbed last year; they won't be able to directly compare their times or match the number of times they climb the building trip for trip.

Twenty-four of us are scheduled to participate in the elite sprint, which begins at 8:00 a.m. I had almost decided not to do the sprint since I've gained about ten pounds and don't think I'll be very fast. It's a short race, though, so I figure I might as well go ahead and do it. What have I got to lose (besides the ten pounds)? As the start time approaches, we head outside and line up. Most of the participants are West Coast Labels/ X-Gym team members, so we trade places with one another in line to allow those we think are faster to go ahead so we don't have to pass one another. As competitive as we are, there is a strong camaraderie among us and everyone is very sportsmanlike—for the sprint, anyway.

They send us off about thirty seconds apart, which is huge. Justin Stewart of Illinois, the favorite, takes off first. His time will be 1:49.2—that's twelve stories in fifty-five seconds, six in twenty-seven-and-a-half seconds, or less than five seconds *per floor*. Absolutely amazing! He finishes twenty seconds in front of PJ and thirty seconds ahead of Jeff Dinkin, both world-class climbers. I finish in nineteenth place with a time of 4:13.4. Considering that I felt like my legs were made of lead and I trudged up the stairs in slow motion, I'm happy with my finish. My time for twenty-five floors the year before was 4:41, so I did improve. In practice I do the ten-story building in about two minutes, so my body's natural adrenaline response gave me a nice little boost to finish in just over double that, not counting the extra floors.

We hang out at the finish for photos; we chat, then stretch and hydrate before the Towerthon begins at nine. There are almost two hundred people signed up to participate in the two-hour climb. We line up in no particular order, except that some of the more competitive runners—including my brother Mark—want to start at the front. Mark and Mike Caviston from Coronado were the top two finishers last year, so they get in front as along with Jeff Dinkin and Justin Stewart. Mark didn't do the sprint this morning. He wants to focus his energies on the multi-climb. I'm back in the line, maybe fifteen or twenty people from the start. The volunteers at the start ask us to note our start time (there's a huge display clock there) so we know when our two-hour time limit is up.

I'm not overly nervous. This is my first time competing in the Towerthon, and I'm not in a hurry. It's more about stamina than speed—at least for me, anyway. The first song on my iPod today is a worship song with a line that says, "I will run and not grow weary." I joke with another climber, Madeleine, that I hope that's true of climbing, too. Several of the guys are really wound up, including one of my male teammates who shall remain unnamed. On the first ascent, at about the tenth floor, he is yelling at a younger girl to move to the right (courtesy dictates that faster runners be allowed to pass on the inside rail), but she isn't paying attention to him. He gives her a shove and brushes her out of the way. This elicits a shocked response from the female volunteer at the landing who is handing out water. She looks at me as if to say, "Wow, did you see that?" I give her a little grin. His action was unsportsmanlike, I must say. I have never seen behavior like that in any other climb I've done, but I chalk it up to testosterone and adrenalin.

Today we're climbing two separate stairwells in the same building. Each is identical, but they have assigned one to competitive climbers and the other to casual climbers. The girl who was pushed aside belonged in the other stairwell. I didn't see her again, so I assume she moved over to the other side after that eventful first trip. Many casual climbers don't realize the many, many hours of rigorous training that competitive climbers put in each week to be the best they can be. To sacrifice so much time and devote so much energy to invest in a race, only to be held up by someone who has no investment and is not even competing, is extremely frustrating.

At the 2012 U.S. Bank Climb, I was stuck in so much "traffic" on the way up that at times I was basically trudging behind six to eight casual climbers, waiting for a chance to pass through. My time the year before was good enough to get me an elite spot, but if I had done that, I would not have had a chance to medal; I'm not fast enough to beat the top women climbers in that race. If a climber enters as an elite, he or she is no longer part of the age group competition, unless the climber registers and pays twice. I've asked the race organizers to consider offering climbs in elite, competitive, and recreational categories to allow for better racing conditions in the stairwells.

Believe it or not my biggest concern going into this climb is sweating. When I did 4,800 stairs the morning of my birthday, I sweated more than I have ever sweated before. I always sweat profusely *after* a run, but that only lasts for a couple of minutes. I know that once I start to sweat in the Towerthon, I'll sweat for the rest of the two hours.

I'm wearing a pair of nylon shorts and a longline sports bra. I don't know at what point I began to sweat, but by the third or fourth trip up, things are heating up. They have a blower on one of the floors, probably halfway up or so. It feels great. My motivation becomes getting to the top, taking the elevator down, and walking outside into the lovely cool air. The high temperature in San Diego is supposed to be in the low seventies today, but right now, it's mid-sixties and heavenly each time I step outside. Volunteers and staff wipe down the interior handrails throughout the climb, which is also extremely helpful. I wear gloves, but many climbers don't, so the rails are slick with sweat. Even with people drying them regularly, by the last few laps they are very slippery, and I lose my grip several times.

I was concerned before the climb that I wouldn't be able to keep track of how many trips I was making, but due to the fact that I have plenty of time to think about it on the way up, I keep track easily. I try not to look up at the floor numbers until I absolutely have to, but for some reason floor eighteen is where I most often do. My silent response is always the same: "Ugh, six more!" Later, in talking with some of my teammates, they mention they did the exact same thing. The eighteenth floor must be where the going gets tough.

This climb is very different from all the other races because we all climb the building over and over. This gives me a chance to meet new people and chat in the stairwell. Some climbers don't like it—it messes with their concentration. For me, though, talking to other people is a welcome distraction in such a solitary sport. In practice I rarely pass anyone in the stairwells, and when I do we seldom exchange words. In a regular race I am way too focused (and out of breath) to say anything unless absolutely necessary. Being able to talk to other people as I climb is fabulous! I talk to one other climber nearly the whole trip up on one leg, and the time passes quickly. On another leg, I see a guy with a WCL/X-Gym shirt on and introduce myself as Mark's sister. He tells me his name is Esteban and says he recognizes me from our Facebook page. Alberto also wears a WCL/X-Gym shirt. He and I pass several times. He's very friendly and is doing great. He tells me how many repetitions he's done, and I ask other climbers how many ascents they've done. Some give me a number, some say they've lost track, and some ignore me, too deep in their "zone" to respond.

At the top volunteers offer Gatorade, water, and pickle juice. I saw pickle juice mentioned on someone's Facebook post regarding this climb and thought it was a brand name of a sports drink, but no—it's actual pickle juice. It's supposed to help with leg cramps. I take a small sip of Gatorade after six or eight trips up and eventually sample a bit of pickle juice. I don't know why I think it might taste differently from what I expected, but it's just your basic pickle juice. Yuck!

Super fit, super fast Tommy Coleman, who owns the seventy-five-story U.S. Bank record of 9:27 (set in 2013), has cracked ribs today, and is unable to compete. He's at the top welcoming us after each trip, saying, "Great job," "You're doing great," and "Keep it up." That means so much to me. PJ and Beverly, who flew down from Seattle just to do the sprint, take positions along the stairs with a camera, snapping photos of us as we pass. They also call out words of encouragement. As I said, since this is such a lonely sport, having them along the way makes the event so much more pleasant. I appreciate their words so much more than I can say.

After several trips, I arrive at the top to find Madeleine curled up in a fetal position in agony with a volunteer rubbing the inside of her thighs.

She has cramps in her quads. I feel terrible for her; I tell her I hope she's okay and head toward the elevator. There are four elevators with a volunteer in each, and other volunteers are busy expediting climbers into the elevator cars and sending them quickly on their way. On several trips I encounter Father Joe operating the elevator. Father Joe, a portly older priest in a wheelchair, heads up the charity that will benefit from today's climb. Each time I see him I ask, "How many is this for you, Father Joe?" and he gives me a number. He's keeping track of his trips up just as we are, and he's way ahead of the rest of us.

One of the elevators has a slight lip where it doesn't quite meet the floor on which it has stopped, so of course I trip over it at least three or four times during the event and feel like an idiot for not watching my step each time I do it. Later several other climbers also mention doing the same thing. Well, at least none of us did a face-plant as far as I know!

It takes me an hour to complete my first eight trips up the building. This is terrific. I really don't have a goal since I have no idea of what to expect or what kind of pace I can keep up, but I'm very happy with my progress. Stan has calculated that eighteen times up is a vertical mile. Mark and Michael did nineteen and twenty times last year (keeping in mind they climbed all twenty-five floors), so I know I am doing a respectable job. In seeing my split times after the race, I slowed down on nearly each consecutive climb. Some of the guys actually got faster on their last couple of trips. Amazing!

After about the tenth ascent, I realize I should've eaten something between the sprint and the Towerthon. I never get hungry while climbing—there's not enough time—but I'm getting fatigued, and I need some fuel. There is a large table in the lobby with bagels and fruit, so as I pass by I grab a quarter of a raisin bagel and eat it quickly while walking back around the building to the entrance. I'm not sure what I'll do next year (yes, I'm doing it again next year!)—maybe I'll carb up the night before, which is normally not necessary with stair climbing since the races are over so quickly.

Climbing with food in my stomach doesn't work for me. I'd eaten a banana before one San Diego climb in the spring and got a stomach ache about half way up the building. As much as my legs and lungs burn during a climb, the last thing this climber needs is one more unhappy body part.

After completing eight climbs in the first hour, I was hopeful I could do sixteen total, but I begin to slow down after the tenth. At this point I start doing single steps and only throw in double steps occasionally when I feel I can. About an hour and forty minutes in, I begin fretting about how many more ascents I can do. My legs are getting tired, and occasionally my toes catch the stair ahead, making me stumble. Whenever I see a guy coming up behind me with a towel over his head, I know it's Mark. He's sweating like crazy and has the towel over his head to catch the perspiration. I had a towel tucked into the front of my top, but by this time I'm carrying it because I'm using it so frequently. At lunch afterward, I notice that the bridge of Mark's nose is rubbed raw from wiping his face so often.

I was worried that the extra ten pounds I was carrying would affect me in the sprint, but it's actually making me work harder with each and every ascent. *Why, oh why, do I eat things I shouldn't eat?* is one thought that repeatedly crosses my mind. Mark, who smokes an occasional cigar, says he asks himself, *Man, why did I smoke that cigar?*

Mostly, I'm occupied with my music and seeing everyone along the way. Toward the end, my competitive instincts rear their little heads and I begin calculating how fast I have to go to complete the last few trips. Before I go in for number twelve, I ask the man at the start how it works as we near the end of our time. He tells me that as long as I enter the stairwell before the end of the two hours, it will count. I have about fifteen more minutes, so know I can get in two more. Now, on the thirteenth trip, I'm doing all double steps again and really working and sweating hard. My legs aren't especially hurting and my lungs aren't burning; instead I'm experiencing a feeling of overall tiredness—just being worn out. I don't know how long the elevator trip takes, but depending on the wait, it has to be close to a minute. Now I'm pushing it. As I enter the stairway for my final lap, I still have about eight or nine minutes. As long as I have a goal, I can do all doubles and pivot on the turns. As I pop out on the top floor, I am very relieved to be finished. I feel such a great sense of accomplishment. I later calculate that I climbed 7,275 stairs. Stan says there are 485 steps, and I did fourteen times that in the 'Thon (6,790) plus 485 more in the sprint. My birthday climb had been a nice warm-up for this event.

I head back down to the lobby where they've already posted results. I'm up there with thirteen, but I know I have one more than that. Other climbers there confirm that you need to add one to the posted totals. I go to the restroom and come back to find Marisol and Imelda, Luis' wife, in the lobby. We wait around for our other teammates, but they never appear. I asked a volunteer if she knows where everyone is, and she tells us they're on the third floor. The three of us ride the elevator up and join the post-race celebration. The organizers provide live music, food, and beverages for everyone in a lovely outdoor courtyard, but most of our team isn't here. We wait, and finally they straggle in. They had been taking team photos upstairs. The three of us are disappointed to find out that we missed out on being included.

Justin was the winner with twenty-six trips, none of which took him more than 3:29. Mark and Scott Stanley, the pride of Texas, had twenty each. Mike Caviston and Jeff Dinkin each had twenty-two. Alberto and another teammate had twenty-one each. Representing the females, Lisa and Cindy Levine each did eighteen. Madeleine and I both had fourteen.

I check the results in my age group and expect to get a medal. As they call out the winners in the age categories, I realize that organizers have sorted us into age groups in twenty-year increments; twenty to forty, forty to sixty, and so on, not the usual ten-year spread, so I do not medal. The reward for this climb would have to be the satisfaction of donating to a very worthy cause and the knowledge that I had done a terrific job for my first time here.

I do the 2014 Towerthon but don't fare as well. Thirty year-old Jason Larsen won the event with twenty-eight repetitions up a building shorter than the one we climbed in 2013. Mark had twenty-four, and I did fifteen. I am cocky and start out very fast. I do my first five trips in less than half an hour, thinking I will smash my 2013 total easily. Instead I completely burn out after the first hour. Fifty-nine-year-old Imelda, Luis's wife, humiliates me by completing eighteen trips. Veronica's mom, seventy-year-old Margarita Stocker, does one more than I do. Slow and steady wins the Towerthon—lesson learned.

CHAPTER FIFTEEN

U.S. Bank Steps, 2013

The climb up the U.S. Bank Tower began in 1993 as an annual event during a series of competitions, including beach volleyball. Until 2004 the September climb cost more for the organization to put on than it raised. The organizers skipped the event in 2005 to research ways to make it profitable. It was worth it.

Today's race has 3,700 registered participants, 3,400 who actually do the climb. It raises $640,000 to benefit many of the Stewart Ketchum Downtown YMCA's community based programs, funding after-school activities, preschool enrollment, health screenings, and summer camps, as well as other youth and family programs. As a result of the events of September 11, 2001, a "High Rise Heroes" division was added to the climb to honor firefighters from surrounding communities. The firefighters climb with about sixty pounds of gear, competing in their own category.

Climbers can compete in elite or individual categories or as a team. Participants must qualify to compete as an elite by meeting time requirements or ranking minimums. The "open" individual category is divided into male and female categories, then into age groups: 20–29, 30–39, and so forth. My brother has competed both as an elite and as an individual. Mark says climbing is "all about the hardware [medals]," so if he thinks he can beat the other elite climbers, he will compete in the elite division. If not, he competes as an individual so he can medal in his age group. Medals are given to the top three male and female finishers in each age group and to the top male and female elite.

Nothing about the day of my sixth U.S. Bank Climb is particularly outstanding except I'm really not in the mood to climb today. I have gained weight and am not feeling particularly fit. My running has been limited to mostly one-and-a-half to two-and-a-half-mile runs five mornings per week. I haven't been making the time to do the longer three- and four-mile runs I did pre-U.S. Bank 2012 that helped me achieve a PR (personal record) of 16:54.

Brantley Watson, a reporter for the *Orange County Register*, had contacted me a couple of weeks ago. He is interested in doing a story about "tower racing," as his editor Roger Bloom calls it. Roger had been the editor of *The Independent*, a small local paper serving a couple of individual beach communities. Newport Beach, where I live, was one of them. Roger had sent a reporter to do a story on me in April 2011 after my fastest overall female finish in Pittsburgh, and he told Brantley about me. Brantley had never heard of competitive stair climbing and was intrigued enough to want to do a piece about me. We arranged to meet in LA at the climb for an interview. I wanted so badly to be in the best shape I could, but I had struggled all summer with my weight and didn't devote the time necessary to be at my best. I'm not confident at all today.

It's a huge event, and my start time is scheduled for around three in the afternoon. The late start poses a problem about what to eat leading up to the race. Early morning climbs are easy: I eat a little something, but there's not a lot of time to think about it. Why didn't I record what I'd eaten last year? Today I eat my usual two egg whites and piece of whole grain toast for breakfast. I skip the salsa, fearing that it will upset my already nervous stomach. I also eat my normal midmorning snack consisting of six ounces of yogurt and an apple.

I leave work around noon to get ready to go to LA. I'm hungry but have no idea what I should eat. I decide on three ounces of leftover grilled chicken. I make a half sandwich of almond butter on whole grain bread to take with me in the car in case I get hungry on the way. I eat it about halfway there. Craig is doing this climb with me and will drive, as usual, so I try to sit back and relax and not obsess about the challenge ahead.

When we arrive, I find Brantley right away and introduce myself. He asks how I am and what my goal is for the climb. I tell him 16:53, a second faster than 2012. I always aim to improve on each climb, but I don't know if I can do that today; I figure even a second faster than last time will be good enough. I introduce Brantley to Mark and a few other teammates. The reporter is fascinated by Mark's knowledge and experience and intrigued by the fact that he built stairs into the hill behind his house so he could train. He is also very impressed by Mark's ranking as one of the top thirty climbers in the world. Brantley ends up splitting the article, featuring stories about both Mark and me.

I head for the locker room to use the restroom before the race. I encounter Veronica and Madeleine who have both already run and had great times. Madeleine says she beat Karen Geninatti, the little power-house from Illinois, in my age group. I say, "Wow, amazing!" Karen is a fierce competitor. Madeleine says Karen told her she had gained seven pounds so that slowed her down. We both burst into laughter because Karen doesn't seem to have a single ounce of extra weight on her tiny, sub-five-foot frame. She is a former bodybuilder, all lean muscle—an amazing athlete.

Madeleine has no idea how much what she just said bolsters my spirits for the climb. I weigh 152.5 today. I've managed to peel off about four pounds, but ideally I'd be at least ten pounds lighter. Every time over the past few months I ate something I knew I shouldn't, I would say to myself, "You know Karen Geninatti isn't shoving a cookie/candy/whatever into her mouth right now. She has willpower!" Madeleine's comment reminds me that we are all human and we each struggle to be the best we can be. Right now that makes me feel a lot better about where I am physically.

On the way to the start, I talk to other teammates who have already finished. Most of them raced as elites. I'm participating in the general climb in order to have an opportunity to medal in my AG. Tommy Coleman has set a new building record of 9:27 and is the overall winner. Last year's winner, Jesse Berg, is on a later flight out of Chicago. He hasn't arrived yet, but the consensus is that he won't beat Tommy's time. Jesse eventually runs it in a little over ten minutes to take second place overall.

As I get ready to queue up, I stretch and get my iPod, earbuds, and gloves in place. All I have to do is squeeze the earbud cord to turn it on as I cross the mat. I take off just after 3:10 p.m. I wear a sports watch and always try to memorize the exact time, but today I am so nervous that all I remember is 3:10 and some seconds. I like the fact that ten is an even number and easy to remember so I can keep track of my pace. I squeeze the cord on my buds and . . . nothing. The music isn't coming on. I try a couple more times, but soon I need to grab the handrails. I'm using a brand-new pair, a gift from my daughter Ariana, and I figure I'll mess with the buds as soon as I get a rhythm going. Once I start climbing, though, I don't want to take a precious second to let go of the handrail and fiddle with them, so I plunge onward, listening only to my labored breathing.

I soon have a bigger problem: I am so thirsty! I haven't been this thirsty in a climb for a very long time. My tongue feels like sandpaper. All I can imagine is that I might swallow it, which is absurd, but so is racing up a tall building. I am literally panting. My tongue seems to have taken on a life of its own; it's wagging to and fro. I'm smacking my lips, and I can only imagine what I must look like with my mouth contorted. I'm mortified. I'm only about fifteen stories up, with a very long way to go. I'll never make it. I accept a cup of water somewhere around floor twenty and hang onto it for about five floors; I don't want to let it go. I take a sip each time I hit a straightaway, even though I know this will cost me time-wise.

Listening to my breathing is torment. I'm gasping for air and still have halfway to go. I turn one corner and see a guy sitting right on the steps. Most people who have to stop will lean against a wall in a corner at a landing, but this guy is sitting right in the middle of the steps. I want to tell him to move but can't muster the energy. I slip past and plod on. My teammate Luis passes me, the only person I recognize who passes me this climb. He teases me by saying something about my being slow, which makes me smile. I start going through all my typical mental stairwell conversations. *This is it—my last climb. I'm never, ever, EVER doing this again. I'm too old for this shit! I'm just walking the rest of it; I don't care anymore. I'm going to stop and take a rest and get my music going. Who cares about my time—I sure don't!*

Then the competitor within me and my inner cheerleader start arguing back. *This is what you do, Jane. You're a stair climber. Just keep going, one step at a time. You're two-thirds of the way.* Then, *Only twenty more!* By this time, I'm struggling to do the math in my head. Somewhere around floor sixty-five, my left calf starts to cramp. I pray it doesn't get worse. Last year I had terrible post-race cramping in both calves, so I've been worried about it happening again. Fortunately these cramps are minor and fit right in with the rest of my overall discomfort. My quads are burning. I can't get enough air, and I literally feel like I may burst into flames. I'm burning up; sweat is running into my eyes. My rubber gloves are of no use in wiping the sweat away; I try to use my forearm, but it takes too much effort.

This is my sixth time up U.S. Bank, so I'm relieved when the stairwell narrows; I know I'm nearing the top. The tough part at this stage is not getting stuck behind a slow climber because it's pretty much impossible to pass anyone—and definitely impossible to pass politely. I don't see anyone ahead, so I push forward as hard as I can, hoping to finish strong. I see a flash as a photographer snaps a picture just before I step out into the lovely fresh air. My wobbly legs carry me to the wall that rims the deck, and I plop down unceremoniously. I check my watch—the time is just 3:27. I calculate that it took me about 16:30. I'm ecstatic! Not only did I beat my 2012 time, this is my new PR for the building.

We've been instructed to get off the roof here rather quickly since it's such a small area up here—basically only a walkway rimming the crown of the building, which has a round cap. I sit for a few moments until I catch my breath and feel like I can walk again. A volunteer standing nearby hands me a participant medal. I thank her and head back down a few floors to a suite where volunteers are serving orange wedges, apples, and bottled water. I grab a bottle of water—all I can think about at this point is how thirsty I am. I use a restroom on this floor and wash my sweaty hands; they get sweaty even inside the gloves. I tell myself this wasn't such a big deal; I need to remind myself not to be so nervous next time. I will always make it to the top; it's just a matter of how long it will take.

I left my phone in the locker room so I can't take any photos. I head down in the elevator. Climbers have to take two or three different elevators to get back down to the ground floor. In the first one, I encounter Craig and a Y volunteer, Melody, who I met during the practice climbs. I introduce her to Craig. She tells him she was the one handing out the participant medals on the roof (everyone gets a medal for completing this climb). I tell her she's not the one who gave me mine. She says yes, she was; she was the only one giving them out. I would've sworn she had a different color T-shirt on and different color hair. I joke that all the blood in my brain apparently went to my thighs during the climb.

When I get to the bottom, I walk around, talk to teammates, go to the locker room, and then sit down to chat with Brantley. I check the app on my iPhone during the interview to see whether my time has posted and it has: 16:28. I am very happy. What was all that worrying about, anyway? I check the times posted on the street after the interview and see that right now I'm first in my age group, but I don't count on staying there. It's early, and there are still hundreds of people yet to climb. What I didn't know at this point is that Lisa Ziegel, who had already climbed as an elite, had registered to climb as an individual also. Even on her second trip up the building that day, Lisa beat me handily with a time of just over fifteen minutes. A woman who I had never heard of placed second, but I hung on to garner a third-place medal. I had only medaled one other time at this building, in 2010, when I placed first in my AG, with a much slower time of 17:22. This has been a very nice climb, indeed.

CHAPTER SIXTEEN

Steps to Willis

Back in June after the Towerthon in San Diego, I decided I would register to climb Chicago's Willis Tower—formerly the Sears Tower, and still commonly referred to as the Sears Tower. It was the tallest building in the world from the time it was completed in 1974 until 1998. At the time of the climb, the 108-story building was the tallest in the United States. The spire on the building at One World Trade Center in New York City, completed in early 2014, makes it taller. The Willis Tower race is always the first Sunday in November, which falls on November 3rd this year.

As the day to fly out approaches, pre-climb doubts, fears, and jitters start creeping into my mind. There are so many other things I could be doing with my time and money than flying halfway across the country to climb a building. I was excited at first. Since I've never climbed Willis before, all I have to do is set a baseline time for comparison if I ever decide to climb it again.

Soon after the towerrunningusa.com rankings were updated to include the U.S. Bank Climb, David Hanley messaged me. He calculates the U.S. rankings and tells me that if I finish Willis in the top sixty-two female climbers, I'll move into the list of top-twenty female climbers in the country. My third place finish in my AG at U.S. Bank moved me up from the number twenty-five spot to number twenty-three. I really wish he hadn't told me this. It makes this climb much more stressful. I was the fifty-fifth female at U.S. Bank, and I believe there will be about the same number of climbers at Willis, so while it is possible for me to finish in the top sixty-two, it'll be tough. I've climbed U.S. Bank six times; this will be my first time at Willis—my first visit to Chicago, as a matter of fact.

My training routine has stayed pretty much the same. I climb three times per week and run one-and-a-half to two miles five mornings per week. I walk a bit over three miles each Monday and do shorter walks with the dogs every day. I weigh in at exactly 150 pounds the morning of my flight to Chicago. I wish I was lighter—it would make the climb a bit easier—but this is as good as it's going to get.

Mark and I are scheduled to fly out of John Wayne airport in Santa Ana Friday morning, November 1st. We had unintentionally booked flights that take off minutes apart on different airlines. He picks me up to take me to the airport. We plan to meet at my gate so we can chat while we wait to board. When Mark gets to my gate, he tells me there's been a shooting at LAX. Three people have been shot, not seriously injured—although we find out later that a TSA agent was killed in the incident. We both get messages on Facebook from concerned step-siblings and messages from teammates now stuck at LAX, which has been shut down. Madeleine and her family stopped for breakfast and just missed being there. She and her husband, Steve, daughter Marisol and son John Henry are all slated to climb Willis. Lisa and Stan and his future wife, Kathleen, are all stranded inside the terminal. They are all contemplating going home and flying out Saturday. What a mess! It's time to board, so I'll have to wait for an update until we arrive in Chicago.

I land at O'Hare at 5:20 p.m. Friday. I've had connecting flights through Chicago in the past, but this will be my first time to the city. O'Hare makes a great first impression. The airport is contemporary and welcoming; the United terminal has a flowing neon light display above the escalators and Gershwin playing in the background. I love it! I make my way to baggage claim and then to the trains. A violinist sits on a stool playing a beautiful melody, something familiar, but I'm a bit disoriented and can't figure out what it is. I buy a train pass and try to phone Mark, but I have no cell reception. He had called just as my plane touched down to say his plane had landed alongside mine; he could see us land on an adjacent runway. I finally see him at the train pass kiosk. Climber Steve Stermer from Colorado Springs is with him; he and Mark spotted one another in the terminal.

The three of us take the train out into the dark, drizzly Chicago weather. Mark and Steve are headed to the Bucktown area of the city to get pizza at a place where Mark had eaten the last time he was here. I'm staying with Lene, a friend of mine who lives in Chicago with her husband and son. She picks me up at the station closest to her home. She offers the guys a ride to nearby Bucktown since it's raining steadily at this point, and they accept. We drop them off and head home. Most of the other members of our team will be going home Sunday after the climb, but I want to stay on to visit and explore the city.

I head downtown Saturday afternoon to check into a hotel before going to our team dinner at Lou Malnati's. Mark has graciously paid for a hotel room nearer Willis for tonight. I check in, then head out to explore. I have about an hour and a half before I need to be at the restaurant. I'm surprised to see so many people in Chicago. I forget that Orange County and LA are not the only crowded areas of the country. I like the feel of this city. My first clue was the employee stationed at the ticket kiosk at O'Hare helping travelers buy their train cards. People are friendly (I ask for directions a couple of times), and there are lots of unique shops and restaurants lining almost every street.

I get to the restaurant shortly after 4:00 p.m. There are about two-dozen climbers there so far. I'm surprised that I don't recognize most of them. Between the climbs and our Facebook page, I expected to see more familiar faces. The restaurant sets large bowls of salad and pasta marinara on the tables, family style, and a banquet table with four or five kinds of Chicago's famous deep dish pizza is off to the side. I have a large serving of salad, no pasta, and two pieces of sausage pizza. I attempt not to eat the entire crust, but I'm starving (and it's very good), so I eat almost every bite. Oz (John Osborn) sits beside me and has only one piece of pizza. Karen doesn't have any—I think she just eats salad. We end up packing the room with at least fifty people, including a couple of spouses and some children. Several of our WCL teammates are still not here yet due to the shooting at LAX. They've missed out on tonight's dinner, and we've missed spending time with them.

After the meal, we have a talent show, organized by Mark. Napoleon Woo kicks it off by presenting Mark with a very good sketch he did of him. Oz made a beautiful etched "West Coast Labels" logo on metal for Mark. A couple of the guys juggle, and then Leland stands up. As he passes by on his way to the front of the room, I ask if he's going to rap, and he smiles. He had posted a rap song on FB several months ago about stair climbing, which was a huge hit with all of us. He incorporated the names of lots of the climbers in the song, but I wasn't mentioned. Tonight, he unveils a new song peppered with our names and I'm delighted to hear my name in the chorus. For once, "Jane" rhyming with "pain" pays off for me. The room roars with approval when he finishes. It's the perfect finale to the evening. We break from the tables, chat a bit, and then head off to try and get some sleep. Most of us will be waking early—we need to get to Willis around 6:00 a.m. the next morning for the 7:00 elite start.

I set my alarm for 5:30 and order a wakeup call just in case. Lisa calls to say she just arrived at her hotel. She recounts her experience at LAX. She stepped off the shuttle and encountered people running and screaming, "Run! He has a gun!" It sounded like something from a movie. One of the men who had been shot in the leg had been scheduled to fly out on the same plane as Lisa. She had been stuck at the airport all day Saturday.

I relax and play games on my iPhone and watch TV until about 10:00 p.m. We have the "fall back" time change tonight, and it couldn't have come at a better time for me. I'll be getting up at 3:00 a.m. California time, so the extra hour's sleep will make it that much easier. I wake several times during the night, most memorably at 3:00 a.m., when I tell myself there's no way I'm going to do the climb; I'm going to simply turn off my alarm and forget about it. I fall back to sleep, wake again at 5:00, and get out of bed.

I do a series of stretches (quad, hamstring, and calf) and roll my legs out with a little rolling pin I brought with me. I shower, put on all my gear, and head downstairs to catch a taxi. The driver is not very friendly, but who can blame him—it *is* 6:00 in the morning. I sit quietly as we drive past lots of people with bibs on. I'm surprised to see so many people heading for the climb already; there must be hundreds of them. I then notice something about "hot chocolate" on the bib, and realize there is a different event going on. I ask the driver, and he confirms there's a huge 5k in town that morning. He asks if that's why I'm here. I tell him I'm going to climb the Willis Tower. He then asks, "The inside or the outside?" Ha! Most people think it's crazy enough that I climb stairwells, but this guy thinks I look like someone who could scale the outside of the country's tallest building! Hilarious. I smile every time I think about his comment.

CHAPTER SEVENTEEN

Stepping Out in Chi-Town

As the taxi pulls up along side the skyscraper, I see people buzzing around inside. Mark is near the entry and has my packet—my bib, timing chip (a strip, actually, like they used to use at U.S. Bank), T-shirt, and some freebies. I have to ask for help putting on the strip—I am so nervous! I check my coat and goodie bag and head for the restroom. I jog around a little bit upstairs to loosen up and get a tissue for the runny nose I've gotten in the cold Chicago weather. I'm praying that my nose doesn't run in the stairwell. Sweating profusely is bad enough. I tell Karen Geninatti that I don't think I can do it. She arches her eyebrows, and with fire in her eyes, tells me that I most certainly can and makes me say "I can do it!" out loud. Yes, ma'am!

Today's climb raises over a million dollars for RIC, the Rehabilitation Institute of Chicago. Their website says they are "the nation's number one-ranked provider of comprehensive physical medicine and rehabilitation care to patients from around the world and . . . the leader in research and development of the most cutting-edge treatments and technologies in its field."

RIC has a hand cycle category at the climb for disabled participants which tests upper body endurance. Stationary hand cycles are calibrated for resistance and time to match the 103-floor stair climbing experience. The area beside the starting line is full of hand cyclists doing their thing.

The time passes quickly, and we begin to line up for the elite start. Team West Coast Labels/X-Gym members are everywhere. I keep scanning the crowd and finally see Madeleine and Lisa, but there's still no sign of Stan. Madeleine had been diagnosed with breast cancer a few weeks ago. She had a partial mastectomy on Wednesday, including the removal of some lymph nodes, but still insists on climbing today. Her doctor told her it was fine as long as she didn't pull with her arms. I understand how important this is to her after what I went through with my knee, but I am worried she might hurt herself. She has climbed Willis before, though, so she knows what to expect.

I let several faster climbers go ahead of me in line—why make them pass me if they don't have to? I begin to worry about my throat and being thirsty, especially after U.S. Bank. I wish I'd brought a cough drop. Karen suggested this after U.S. Bank; she told me keeps one in her cheek during climbs, and it helps her. Just as I think it, Harish, who I met for the first time at dinner the night before, offers me a cough drop. Perfect, providing I don't inhale it and choke to death in the stairwell. I pop it in my cheek a few seconds before I get the go-ahead to climb. My goal is to finish in less than thirty minutes. I calculated on paper that I should be able to do it several minutes faster, but this race ain't run on paper!

Thankfully the start is inside, since it's cold outside. Before I know it, it's time to go. I take off at 7:06 a.m. I run about fifteen feet through a doorway; the first of Willis' 2,115 steps are off to the left. I was warned on Saturday night that the rise of the steps is very steep. Boy, they weren't kidding. I'm focused on the step pattern I had worked out with David Hanley, but the first few flights contain a strange number of steps, so it's not working very well so far. Several climbers barrel around me. I sure don't know how anyone could keep up that pace for a 103 floors, but I don't have the energy to worry about them. Soon the stairs do come in sets of ten. Single step right foot, double, double, double, double, single onto the landing with my left foot, pivot and repeat. Wow, they are so *steep*. I wish I had been practicing on bleachers—bleachers are higher than typical steps. I feel like my legs would be adjusting better if I had; my short stubby legs aren't providing much "spring." I don't look up to see what floor I'm at until somewhere in the high twenties. Even then, the numbers are not right out in plain view; they're tucked around the corner. This is good; I don't want to be tempted to look up continuously.

Volunteers offer water. I ignore them. Some call out how far we are ("You're 29 percent of the way!" was my favorite). I come around weird walls, almost like doorways, and pray that there will be a straightaway around the corner so my quads will get some relief. No such luck. Now as I reach for the handrail, I jam my fingers—there's not enough space; the handrails are too close to the wall. This gives me something else to focus on. It happens several more times—ouch! Doggone it, isn't this already painful enough? Madeleine tells me afterward that she broke off some fingernails inside her gloves because of the tight hand space.

I'm not having too much trouble breathing; I'm not going fast enough. My legs feel tight. Somewhere near halfway up the building, the stairwell switches from right turns to left. I try to adjust my step pattern and manage to do okay; I just wish my legs would go faster. I check my watch—I am a little over eleven minutes. I can't really think, but I figure twice that is twenty-something, and I should be nearing the hundredth floor at that point. If I can keep this pace, I will finish in well under thirty minutes. But as I get up around the high fifties, I start to fade. Having done the seventy-five-story U.S. Bank Climb six times, I've counted on being good at least that far. I look up at sixty-two and think to myself, *I'm done. I* feel sad that all my training hasn't made me feel stronger or faster. I am also so very hot.

I wonder if I could get my jersey off while I climb—I want to rip it off so badly but know I won't. It gives me something to focus on, though. I start single stepping because I'm wobbly. I am shaking as I reach out to grab the handrail, and sometimes I almost miss it. I'm afraid I'll miss it and fall backward, though I'm probably leaning too far forward into the stairs for that to happen. Lisa tells me after the climb that the guy in front of her at one point did just that. She pushed him from behind to keep him from toppling over backward. My throat is fine, though. My mouth is a bit sticky from the sugar in the cough drop, but it's better than being thirsty.

This is the point where I start bargaining with myself. *Do single steps to sixty-five, then doubles to seventy,* I tell myself. After that, I throw in doubles every few steps. I think about the people who have donated to my climb. I think about Darlene Zschech's message about finding my "roar" at the Imagine women's conference at church the night before I left. I tell myself that I am strong; this is what I train to do. *One step at a time.* I remind myself how much difference one second makes, and I go back to doubles.

Around floor eighty-eight, the stairs go into three sets of seven each, and they don't seem to be so steep. I like this a lot; I have hope now. I do one single step, then three doubles, land and repeat. The volunteers are yelling encouragement, "Fifteen more to go, ten more to go, five more to go." Finally I hear the cheers above me, which means the finish is just ahead. I'm going to make it! I say, "Praise Jesus" out loud—which is not very loud at this point since I don't have much breath left in me. I look up for the photo, try to smile, and cross the orange timing mat. There is applause, and I get a participant/finishers medal. I step out into a large carpeted room full of people. I don't look for familiar faces at this point; all I care about is an empty space on the floor. I see one, stagger over, drop down onto my butt and lean against the wall. Oh, thank God, it's over!

I am shaking and sweat-soaked, but also euphoric because I am so relieved. It's difficult to communicate how I feel when I reach the end of a climb like this one. At the beginning, it seems so impossible that I will ever get to the top. During the climb, I feel like I'm moving in slow motion and the stairs will never end. The ascent seems to take place at a snail's pace; it makes crossing the finish line so very sweet. I had checked my watch as I hit the mat and now calculate that I did it in about twenty-five minutes. I am extremely happy. Mostly happy it's behind me, but also very pleased to have easily beaten my goal of thirty minutes.

Now is the fun part. I grab a bottle of water to begin to rehydrate. I spend at least an hour on floor 103. We take lots of photos (some out on the clear Lucite ledges that suspend you over thin air), congratulate one another, and share stories of injuries and victories. I meet Paul Wimbert, who I had seen at the dinner the night before. He tells me that he read about my birthday climb on Facebook and says I inspired him to do five thousand steps on his fiftieth birthday. That means so much to me! I talk to a young man wearing the same gloves I wear. He has come from Philadelphia to climb Willis. What a terrific guy! Leland offers to pay for a SkyDeck photo of the team, so twenty-six West Coast/X-Gym team members jam together on one of the glass platforms for a photo. I'm scared to death. It's supposedly safe up to ten thousand pounds, and someone calculates that we weigh about half that, but it's still very unsettling to stand on a clear surface suspended 103 stories above the ground with that many people. I hang onto the frame with one hand, as if that would make a difference. I pose for more photos with different groups of teammates and finally head to the elevator for a remarkably quick ride to the bottom.

Once down, I see the "results" table. I punch my bib number into a computer and a little piece of paper pops out with my time. I did it in 25:01. Of course, that pesky second would be there to remind me that a couple more double steps would indeed have made a difference. Next time I'll better it. Mark finishes sixteenth overall with a time of 16:43. He's amazing.

I roam around looking for familiar faces and run into Stan, who has completed his first climb and is now contemplating climbing the building a second time if he can find some notepaper and a pen. He wants to double-check the stair count and measure the step height. I tell him he's insane.

Steve Stermer and Steve Ronk say they'll go up with him. I say I'm not going. I tell them the only way I would consider climbing it again is if the stairwell is clear; I don't want to interfere with other climbers. They say we'll be climbing faster than most of the climbers in the stairwell at that point, but I doubt I will be.

Stan finds a yellow pad, a pen, and a piece of cardboard to measure the step height. At some point, I agree to go again. Oh, man, this is nuts. We see Syd. He and Karen have already done a second trip. Steve Ronk backs out to tend to his wife and kids, who want to leave. Steve Stermer, Stan, and I have our photo taken together while we wait in line. We're there for quite a while, and I almost back out. It's 9:45 a.m., and I have to check out of the hotel on the other side of town by noon. But it's too late to change my mind now—we're back at the starting line. The guy there doesn't look very happy at our going in again, but he lets us walk in together at about 9:53 a.m. We take it nice and easy, stopping every ten or twenty floors for a few moments so Stan can measure or jot down notes. Justin Stewart (today's winner with a time of 13:29 by three seconds over a German competitor) passes us by. He's on his third trip up. We hear later that he climbs the building five times, which means he climbed 10,575 stairs.

The second trip proves to be very interesting. I pass signs on the wall saying we've climbed as high as the Eiffel Tower and the Empire State Building. I never saw them the first time. I thank the volunteers for their encouragement. I touch the backs of a few disabled climbers struggling to go one slow, painful step at a time. We pass at least three climbers who have arm or leg braces and helpers assisting them.

I learn later that one of those climbers was Illinois Senator Mark Kirk who suffered a major stroke in January of 2012. He climbed thirty-seven floors in 2012, and this year he manages to climb forty-one. Seeing these climbers has a very sobering effect on me. What courage and determination they have! I am humbled by their efforts. I feel like a whiney crybaby for being afraid of this climb. I so admire each one of the climbers who had to overcome severe physical limitations to climb today. They are the true winners here this morning.

Mark Block of Ankeny, Iowa, is also one of the climbers I pass the on second trip, but I don't know it at the time. He first participated in the hand cycle category in 2010 using only one arm. Mark had been paralyzed as a result of a car accident in the '80s. He walked out of the hospital six months after being told he would never walk again. He suffered a setback in 2009, when he fell and sustained a traumatic brain injury. Mark has climbed to the top of the Willis Tower, one agonizing step at a time, every year since 2011. He has gone on to conquer dozens of other structures in the interim, including Chicago's John Hancock Building. Karen helps Mark as a "spotter"—she climbs beside him to help him focus and protect him from other climbers. What an inspiration this man is!

There's no pressure this trip, but that doesn't stop us from getting hot and sweaty. I am soaked with sweat. Steve and Stan are both dripping wet.

I see that Stan's piece of cardboard is wet with sweat where he's holding it. We comment on different twists and turns and what we were thinking the first time up. There are a couple of strange little floors in the middle and only one "straightaway"—and not much of one, either—where the stairwells change direction. Steve says he wishes he felt this strong the first time up, and says he might even do a third trip. We make it back up to 103 in about thirty-three minutes. I had wanted to take a photo in front of the giant 103 on the wall facing the elevator, but I didn't see it until I was already in the elevator the first time. Now I have a second chance to snap a few pictures there before we head back down.

Steve and Lisa decide to go for round three, and I head out to walk back to my hotel. I learned later that the officials cracked down on those of us doing multiple climbs and stopped Lisa and Steve from going up again. Lisa played the "I got trapped in LAX due to the shooting" card and the woman finally let her through. Organizers no longer permit multiple climbs, so I'm glad I got to do it twice my first time.

In hindsight Willis wasn't all that scary. Knowing what I know now, I will practice on bleachers if I do it again. The step height really made a difference. I also need to work on my upper body strength. Stronger arms would have helped a lot, given the steepness of the stairs. Mark is rowing to improve his climbing. I can do some swimming and resistance work to train for next time, and maybe some weight lifting. *If* I do it again.

CHAPTER EIGHTEEN

Stepping into the Stratosphere

Next I decide to tackle the Stratosphere Hotel Climb in Las Vegas in March, which will benefit the American Lung Association. The distinctive Stratosphere tower resembles the Space Needle in Seattle and rises high above the Las Vegas strip. It's the tallest structure west of the Mississippi, with 108 "levels." I'm not sure how they determine the number of levels, but the stair count is very similar to the AON Building in Los Angeles. AON has 1,393 stairs, and the Stratosphere has 1,391. Knowing this makes the challenge a bit less daunting.

I drive to Vegas Saturday morning for the Sunday climb. One of my clients arranges for me to stay at Hotel 32 in the Monte Carlo. I don't mind not being right at the Strat; getting around Vegas will be easy since I have my car. Saturday evening, we have a mixer at the restaurant on the 107th level of the tower. Thanks to heavy rains in the area earlier in the day, visibility is now clear for miles and miles, and the views are spectacular. I see many familiar faces: Cindy and Kyle Levine, PJ, Karen and Z. It's crowded up here and not ideal for a group, so after a while, more than twenty of us leave and meet downstairs in the hotel to eat. I get to know Maggie Lonnergan and Sherri and Steve Breese better over dinner, as well as Alex Workman. Alex is a world-class climber who typically doesn't venture this far west for climbs, but this climb serves as the U.S. Stair Climbing Championship.

Steve Breese is not happy that the menu doesn't include any "paasta" (pronounced with his Chicago accent), so he orders a baked potato stuffed with another baked potato filled with sour cream, chili, and cheese over a bed of chili! Most of us order salads, but Steve carbs up. I joke that I wouldn't be able to get out of bed if I ate that, let alone climb the building the next morning. It just goes to show how different we all are.

The morning of the climb, my teammate Lisa and I drive over to the Strat and join up with everyone for the start. It's cool and sunny, the perfect morning for a climb. We head inside to line up in the hallway. The jockeying for position starts now, but as usual, there's plenty of bantering back and forth.

"You go before me; I haven't been training that hard."

"No, you're faster, you go ahead."

"I've gained weight."

I settle in between Leland and Nelson. Nelson's injured knee is giving him problems today, so he lets me go ahead of him.

As competitive as we are, there are strong bonds between the members of our "step-family." At a San Diego climb a couple of years earlier, a photographer at the finish line herded members of the West Coast Labels team together for a team photo. As he prepared to snap the photo, he said, "Pretend that you like one another." That elicited groans, giggles, and responses of "*What?*" and "We LOVE each other!" The smiles were genuine in that photo—no pretense necessary.

I've been warned that this building has flights of twenty stairs, which is very different from most. Cindy Levine says she thinks I'll like it, because there are fewer turns. They have also told me that this stairwell is open, which means there are no walls—if you look over the side, you can see all the way down. It sounds scary, but I did like this a lot. I found it to be less restrictive, less "claustrophobic" than most stairwells. And who has time to look down when you're racing up?

I take off and start up. Again, since I have never done this race, there is less pressure because my time will just serve as a baseline for future climbs. My earbuds are working great, I'm listening to terrific music, and I am determined not to look up at the floor numbers until I absolutely can't help myself. I first look up at level forty-three and think, *Wow, that's almost halfway; this is great.* That soon digresses into *Oh lordy, twenty more.* This becomes my mantra. Every time I go around a turn, I look ahead and mutter, "Twenty more." I think the stairs will never end. This climb has volunteers posted as monitors at several places throughout the climb; they speak to me, but I'm in a zone and ignore them. Finally one man repeatedly yells at me, and I realize he wants me to take out my earbuds, so I do. Some climbs prohibit earbuds; they are thought to be a safety hazard because anyone wearing them might not to be able to react in case of emergency.

The only climber I pass on my way up is Leland. When I do, I say, "I'm sorry, I'm sorry" as I pass him on a landing. Toward the top, the stair count mercifully gets shorter, maybe only nine or ten steps to a flight. As I reach the top, I see people and say, "This is it?" just to be sure. One of them gives me a wry smile. Hey, after all that climbing the last thing I want to do is slow down right before hitting the mat. I later view a video of the finish, and when I cross the mat, I let out a big sigh. It wasn't exactly a sigh of relief—more like "Good grief!"

Alex Workman finished second overall with a time of 7:56, behind one of our German dinner companions, Gorge Heimann, who finished with 7:19. Steve Breese finished twentieth overall with a time of 9:41 just behind Mark with 9:35. He beat his salad-eating wife by eight seconds; Sherri was second fastest female overall. I was 141st overall with a time of 14:21.

Leland approaches me in the recovery area where there is food and drink. He says I didn't have to apologize for passing him. I know I didn't, but I could tell during the race that he was hurting, and I know how hard it is. He has since beaten me on at least two occasions, so I'm feeling much better now about having passed him that day.

I get invited to the 2015 Strat Climb as an elite climber because I am ranked 16th female in the nation at the end of the 2014 season. I am struggling with my weight (it still isn't easy after all I've gone through) and am at least fifteen pounds heavier than I was for the 2014 climb. I've been running steadily and going to the AON practice climbs to train. The Tuesday before the race, I climb AON from floor four to fifty-five three times in a little over an hour. I barely make it up the third time and would have quit if I'd been able to get out of the stairwell, but we're in the building after hours and all the doorways are locked off. I am wringing wet with sweat by the time we leave to go to a kick-off party, but I am very glad I got in a strenuous workout.

Saturday morning, Mark and his son Torrey and I road-trip it to Vegas for the climb. I do not sleep well the night before the race. My mind won't turn off. *Why did I have decaf after dinner? I should have had herbal tea. I think that decaf had more than the usual amount of caffeine in it. The pillow is too fluffy; I should have brought my own.*

Then the little angel and devil of competition appear, one at each ear. The angel whispers "You're going to do great; give it your best effort. That's all that you can do, and it will be good enough." The demon tells me that I'm going to embarrass myself by doing poorly, so I should take it easy and walk up. "Why push yourself?" he says. "You're old and chubby—just walk it and forget about your time." I'm tormented by thoughts like this for at least an hour. Earlier in the evening, Mark said that one of the climbers was so stressed about how he would do that Mark suggested he do the climb without a timing chip. Then he could just enjoy the climb without worrying about his time. I seriously consider that option just to quell the extreme stress I'm feeling.

A couple of years ago at the November CF Climb, I told Craig when we were getting out of our cars that I didn't know how long I could keep climbing because the stress was so terrible. We ran into Jeannie a few minutes later and she said the same thing almost word for word. For me, prerace stress is not as much about disappointing my teammates and Mark as it is about disappointing myself. I know each shortcut I've taken in training, each thing I've eaten that I shouldn't be eating, and anything I've done that might cause me not to be as fit and ready for a competition as I could be. It would be nice to get to a place mentally where I don't feel so much pressure. I'm still working on that.

Finally I fall asleep. The next morning, I get to the Strat about fifteen minutes before the 8:00 a.m. start, giving me just enough time to check in and make a last-minute trip to the ladies' room. I run outside and get in line to enter the building. We climb several sets of metal stairs and someone jokingly asks if it's over. We enter a long hallway with a right turn leading to a doorway that houses the bottom of the stairwell. There is a very cold draft, so those of us near the end of the line are shivering.

We order ourselves as best we can from fastest to slowest; I am at the end of the elite fast group. Ahead of me is Dan Dill, who is very fit and trim this season; Leland, also very fit this year; Bob Toews; and most of our team. I see Sarah Johnson and Javier Santiago Garay in a group behind me. Javier is one of the top climbers in the world, and Sarah is also world-ranked. I tell them to go ahead of me. Javier says no and Sarah says she's injured. I tell her that, even injured, she's faster than I am.

We wait for a very long time, it seems. I chat with several climbers around me and meet several new people. Michael Rolhaus is here from New Jersey, two other climbers are from Seattle, and a few are from Southern California. It comes down through the line that the reason we are backed up is because a volunteer struck his head and has to be brought down the stairwell. The open stairway runs up through a shaft in the building with very limited access, so he cannot be taken to an elevator, but instead must be carried down.

Those of us in the ice-cold hallway move up to an alcove to the left around the corner where it's much warmer. I see Cindy Levine there along with several climbers from Mexico. We joke that it will feel good to get hot and sweaty in the stairwell.

Finally the line begins to move. I ask what time it is. The battery in my sports watch was dead when I picked it up to pack it. Mark gave that to me for my fiftieth birthday, so the battery lasted for nearly eight years. It's 8:44 a.m.—we have been waiting here for nearly forty-five minutes.

Soon I'm next in line. I've had my Ricola cough drop in my hand this whole time, wrapping and unwrapping it because of nerves, and now I pop it in my cheek. I get the go ahead and begin to climb. I hit the familiar flights of twenty stairs and settle into a steady pace. I pass a few climbers, and some pass me as I move to the outside of the stairwell to let them go around me. I love this stairwell; I'm able to grip the rails on both sides to help propel me forward faster. I notice Sarah Johnson behind me after a few floors. I tell her to let me know if she wants pass me. I'm waiting for her to make her move. Again this year, I look up for the first time around level forty-five. A speedy climber passes me, and I say "Good job, Michael," mistakenly thinking it's Michael Karlin. This guy looks a lot like Michael.

Now Sarah is at my heels. She is making me go faster, and I hate it. As I hit the next landing, I think I'll just stop for a few seconds, but that pesky Sarah is right behind me, and this forces me to keep going. I start single stepping most steps, and Sarah soon catches me. She puts her foot on the same step I have my foot on, which motivates me to resume double stepping and give it all I have. I'm not much of a moaner or groaner, but now I do groan out loud a couple of times. My stomach hurts from pushing so hard. I manage to stay just ahead of her, and eventually we hit the final short series of steps. Sarah, who is still so close that I can see her arms coming out from behind me on my home stretch photo, says, "Almost there!" I start looking at the level numbers but can't remember if we race to 107 or 108. I think to myself that I've never gone face down at the finish, but this will be the time I do; I'll never be able to walk once I cross the mat. I see 107 ahead and more stairs above, so I know now the race ends on 108. I double step it up the final two flights, hit the mat, and drag my stumpy legs a few feet to plop down on the floor alongside a guy sprawled out, trying to catch his breath. We are both gasping for air. The guy on the floor and I exchange a look, but it takes a few seconds before we can catch our breath enough for a quick "hello." I panic for an instant and think I'm going to hyperventilate, but after a couple more breaths, I relax, and my breathing gradually returns to normal.

I stand up after a few moments and get half a glass of orange juice. I walk around to talk to some of the climbers. I introduce myself to today's winner, Sproule Love from New York City (7:22), and Stephen Marsalese (9:05), who I had mistakenly called Michael on the way up. I apologize to him for that—they really do resemble one another. Scott Stanley (10:10) is there, too. Mark was 26th overall with a time of 10:14, forty-five seconds off his 2014 time.

I mingle for a bit, get my participation medal, and head downstairs to the theater on the second floor of the casino. Organizers have placed four cameras in the stairwell so viewers can watch climbers along the way and at the finish. I see a crowd of people gathered around a table in the lobby area and realize the times are posted there, rolling by on a wall display. I see my time of 14:57. I'm disappointed—that's thirty-six seconds slower than last year. I am 193rd overall, sixty-second among female climbers. Sarah, forty-five, beat me by nine seconds with a time of 14:48.

She tells me with a grin that she was standing next to two guys in their twenties when their times came up, and they were both five minutes slower than the two of us. We giggle. She says we should go stand by them and talk about our times really loudly. I crack up. My time would've been so much slower without her; she forced me to go as fast as I could. She said I helped her, too, and she hoped that her being on my heels hadn't bugged me too much. I tell her that she bugged me in exactly the right way. I'm grateful that she was behind me; the pain has been forgotten.

The only other time this happened to me was at the 2013 CF Climb in Los Angeles. I found myself behind Michael Carcieri in the early part of the race. Every time he started to get ahead of me, I pushed forward to catch up. This happened the entire way up the fifty-three-story building (this race used to be fifty-one stories, but now it ends on the roof). He'd get ahead by half a flight; I'd close the gap to within a few stairs. When we finished on the roof, he ran over to me and thanked me repeatedly. He was so excited. He said I helped him get a great time by pushing him. The more I thought about it, I realized he had helped "pull" me up the building by forcing me to keep up with him. It's difficult to orchestrate this kind of pacing, but when it happens, it's great for both climbers.

As we mill around waiting for the awards ceremony, I meet climbing legend Hal Carlson, who is currently ranked number one in the male 60–69 AG nationally on towerrunningusa.com. He came in twenty-fourth overall today, with a time of 10:02. He always wears a distinctive red-and-white striped vest, which makes me think of a basketball official. He did the Empire State Building Climb this year in 15:03, also twenty-fourth overall. Hal tells me I must introduce myself to Ned Greene.

I find Ned Greene and introduce myself. I always start with "Hi, I'm Jane, Mark's sister"—everyone knows Mark. Ned is a diminutive man, but a giant in stair climbing. He's currently number one in the 70–79 AG and number twenty-eighth male climber in the country. At age seventy, weighing 113 pounds (I haven't weighed 113 since I was eleven!), he zips up any building he tackles. He inspires younger climbers (especially Leland) to stay active and healthy now so they can be like him someday.

CHAPTER NINETEEN

Climbing One WTC, New York City

Mark tells me that there might be a climb at the World Trade Center in New York in 2015. I tell him I'd love to do it. One Monday afternoon in late March 2015, he calls to tell me they just announced the Freedom Tower Climb. I am driving when he calls and the reception is awful; I lose him a couple of times, so the conversation gets chopped up. I ask when it will be, and Mark says May 17. That's less than seven weeks away! I tell him it's too soon. I'm not in good shape, and there's not enough time for me to get ready, so I'm not going to go.

Mark calls me several times over the next two days to give me the latest info on the climb. It will be limited to the first thousand climbers to register. Climbers will climb to the ninetieth floor, and the climb will benefit a foundation set up to honor a firefighter killed on 9/11. I cave by Wednesday; I call Mark at lunch to tell him I'm in. The fact that this is the inaugural climb makes it too exciting to pass up. I've never been to New York and I have extra vacation time I can use to make it a fun trip. If I climb slow, I climb slow. I tell myself this climb is *so* not about me.

I go online and sign up that night. It's expensive, a hundred dollars just to register, with an additional $250 fund-raising required. That's more than double the average climb. Proceeds will benefit first responders and the military.

The Stephen Siller Foundation is sponsoring the climb—officially called the Tunnel 2 Towers Tower Climb, or T2TT Climb. Thirty-four-year-old Stephen Siller, a firefighter, lost his life in the 9/11 attack on the Twin Towers. He had just gone off duty in Brooklyn the morning of the attack and was on his way to play golf with his brothers when he heard over a scanner that a plane had hit the first tower. He headed back to the station but was unable to drive through the gridlocked Brooklyn Battery Bridge. He strapped on his sixty pounds of gear and ran nearly two miles to Tower One, where he died when the building collapsed.

This inaugural climb also honors Captain Billy Burke, another first responder who gave his life in service to others on 9/11. Burke was the only firefighter from his station to die at the Twin Towers. He ordered his crew out of Tower Two when Tower One collapsed, but then stayed behind to assist a man and his wheelchair-bound friend. When Billy's men radioed that they were coming back for him, he repeatedly told them, "Keep going; I'm right behind you." These words are inscribed on the participant medals climbers will receive.

I am nearly twenty pounds heavier than I was when I climbed the 103-story Willis Tower in 2013. One WTC is 104 floors, but we will be climbing only ninety. (No one but stair climbers can use the word "only" in front of "ninety-stories" without sarcasm). The stair count is 1,968 or 1,970. We don't have an official Stan Schwarz count; Stan will not be traveling to New York City for the climb.

I amp up my running and throw in some extra stairs throughout the week. What I really need to do is get back to my strict eating regimen, but I am really struggling with eating sugar. I have been spending too much time on the computer and not enough time hitting the pavement running and, more importantly, walking. I have some good days with sugar and some not so good, but I regain some control and soon feel better about my fitness than I did in March.

I post a fund-raising tool a couple of times on Facebook and raise over a hundred dollars toward the $250 minimum. My friend Ginny, who I've known since we were freshmen in high school, joins me for dinner one night a few weeks before the climb. When I tell her about it, she jumps on the bandwagon and pledges to donate. She then gets three other friends to also contribute, for a total of $125. Two more people donate through Facebook the week before the climb, and I receive my largest donation after the climb. I end up with $485 in donations, well exceeding my fundraising goal. A total of forty-six West Coast Labels/XGym team members sign up for the climb. Together we collect more than $26,000, making us the number one fund-raising team.

I am so nervous the week preceding the climb that I can barely sleep. I beat myself up over and over for gaining weight. I swear it's easier to suffer through being hungry than it is to gain weight and then torment myself over it. But I'm a glutton for punishment. This was my "MO" in the past. I'd do the wrong thing and then berate myself over and over for it. I need to overcome this behavior.

To make matters worse, I put in a request for five days off of work surrounding the climb so I can fly back and stay in the city for a few days. I didn't realize that two of my coworkers had already requested the same dates for family weddings. As a result, I'll have to take a red-eye out on Friday night for the Sunday morning climb. I can't sleep on planes, so this will be interesting.

Beginning Wednesday night, I am very emotional, on the verge of tears. Just talking about the climb is emotional, representing the tragedy of 9/11 and the inherent patriotic aspects. It's going to be a long, difficult climb, and I'm not going to be as fast as I want to be because of the extra weight I'm carrying. As Ariana and I walk the dogs before she takes me to the airport Friday, we run into some neighbors, and I start to cry when I tell them I'm flying out to do the climb. Good grief. I should have had a good cry Thursday night and gotten it out of my system.

My flight leaves Orange County at 9:15 Friday night. I doze on and off, but every time my head falls forward, I wake myself up. About halfway through the flight, I finally nod off for at least forty-five minutes. We arrive forty-five minutes ahead of schedule in Newark at 4:45 a.m. Lisa and Jeannie have taken a similar flight out of LAX. I take the train to Penn Station, followed by the subway to the WTC station. As I exit the station, I see the new Freedom Tower on my left. It's beautiful, gleaming pale blue and dwarfing everything around it. The base is closed off due to construction, at least on the station side. The hotel is only a third of a mile away, but I end up going the wrong way and end up walking about a mile to get there; with all the construction around Ground Zero, it's a bit confusing. My early morning stroll leads me through Battery Park where I'm thrilled to catch my first glimpse of the Statue of Liberty across the river. I hadn't expected to like New York, but the city has made a great first impression. I already love it.

As I approach the hotel, a big black SUV pulls up alongside with a driver who honks the horn repeatedly. I turn around to see what's going on, but the windows are tinted and I can't see inside. A door pops open and I hear someone yelling "Jane! Jane!" It's my teammate Lisa. She and Jeannie have taken a limo from JFK, and we all arrive at the hotel at the same time. Lisa and I are rooming together, but only Jeannie's room is ready this early, so we stash our luggage in her room and head out in search of food. We go to a little shop on the corner for breakfast, and it begins to rain hard. Our teammates David Hanley and Brady Renshaw join us. It's wonderful seeing them—like family getting together. Over the next several hours more step-sibs arrive; we see old friends and meet new ones as well.

A woman Mark and I went to grade school with in Vinco is a travel agent and has booked much of the team rooms at the Holiday Inn near the WTC. She has arranged a reception for us on Saturday night at the restaurant adjacent to the hotel. A group of us take a ferry to the Statue of Liberty and Ellis Island and get back about 2:30 p.m. I nap for thirty minutes before heading to the reception.

At the reception I meet the legendary Dan Akerman, here from Switzerland, and Martin Pederson from Denmark. I can't say it often enough: Stair climbers are the nicest people on the planet, and these two world-class athletes are no exception. Being around my teammates is so invigorating. The conversation mostly revolves around the announcement that we will not be allowed to bring any electronics into the building with us, not even a watch. Phones and iPods are one thing, but not being able to use a watch really has everyone abuzz since many climbers use their watches for pacing. The story is that organizers do not want anything that could be used as a triggering device brought into the stairwell.

Mark arrives later with my bib and climb T-shirt. I'm assigned number 895. I joke on Sunday morning that I'm "$8.95 for today, and today only," but I'm the only one who thinks it's funny. Mark also gives me a sleeveless running bra that I had mailed to him to have silkscreened with the WCL/ X-Gym logo. I am so excited! I've been wearing the same short-sleeved team jersey for years—I want something cooler to wear for this climb.

Being around so much positive energy wipes away my stress, and I get seven hours of sleep before waking early to prepare for the climb. I have a cup of black decaf coffee and a strawberry Greek yogurt ($3.00 from a nearby store—yikes!) for breakfast.

Firefighters and police are up first at 8:00 a.m. Most of us are scheduled in the second wave at 8:10. There is an opening ceremony planned for 7:15, so we all hoof it across from the WTC to a closed-off street where a platform has been set up with a piano and sound equipment. Hundreds of people gather to hear impassioned speeches from the organizers and brothers of the two fallen firefighters. FDNY bagpipers, the New York Tenors, and a father-daughter duo perform. I doubt anyone leaves with a dry eye. The press interviews Madeleine. A Spanish language station interviews Javier and Maria, here from Mexico City. This is all so special. I am very, very happy I decided to participate.

Now down to business. We walk back to One WTC en masse, where we pass through two security checks before queuing up. The second security check includes a pat down. This is definitely not your usual stair climb.

I realize I have to use the toilet. Great. I thought I'd have time to run back to the hotel, but I do not. They have four porta-potties set up, which is not nearly enough; there is a long line. I don't have a choice though, so I'll be carrying my food from last night along with me on the climb. Definitely not ideal.

When I get back in line, there is a huge crowd. I'm used to being in the first batch of runners. One of our teammates, Ariel, finds us and tells we're supposed to be closer to the start, so we gather all the WCL people we can find and move forward. There's one more security screening with metal detectors and then the start.

None of us knows what to expect. This is a first-time climb for everyone. I pop a Ricola cough drop into my cheek. The starter scans my bib to record my start time and says, "Good luck," and I realize I'm supposed to go. This is different, because we normally run across a mat. He waves a paddle over my bib to scan my number instead. I run up to the building and make a left into a doorway. The stairwell is spotlessly clean, light and bright. The handrails are about ten feet apart. I'm terrible with distance, but they're way too far apart to double rail it, which is disappointing.

I get a good rhythm going and am double stepping it. I am almost a little too relaxed now. For some reason, at this moment, I don't feel the anxiety and immediacy of other climbs. Before we left the hotel, I started to get butterflies. I told myself there is nothing difficult about what I'm doing. All I need to do is put one foot in front of the other and repeat, repeat, repeat. I know it's going to be a long climb, so I focus on each flight.

There is staff in wearing suits and ties positioned every other flight or so on the landings (it's a very roomy stairwell), and I wish each one of them a good morning. Somewhere about a third of the way, a couple of much younger men come up behind me. They are breathing very heavily and, erratically, and not hugging the rail. I tell them to grip the rail, relax, take regular breaths, and they will be fine. I tell them "I'm an old lady; I'm going to be fifty-nine on Friday—come on and pass me up!"

"Let's go, let's go, let's go!" I say to at least one other guy behind me. At floor sixty-four, I hear some wiseguy telling everyone there are "sixty-four more." When he says that to me, I say, "I have a finger for you," and tell him there are not sixty-four more floors and to stop saying that. I'm sure he thought he was hilarious, but no one I talked to afterward thought he was one bit funny.

I hear Ariel about two flights ahead of me taking big, loud, gasping breaths. I know he's going at about the same pace as I am because I hear him for most of the trip. He had started fast and passed me early on, so unless he fades, he will beat me. I tell myself that most people can't do what I'm doing, that I should not to be too upset about being a slow poke. Sweat is flying off me; I see it hit the concrete steps and make splash marks. That dang East Coast humidity! I am mostly single stepping now, throwing in doubles as often as I can.

When I see floor eighty-five, I say, "Thank God," and start doing all doubles, counting to myself. I count, "One, two, three, four—nine"; (there are nine more flights to go). I continue, "One, two, three, four—eight," until I get to "one." I push myself up the last flight. As I get to the top, I yell, "Where is the mat?" I'm told it's out and to the left down the hall. *Oh, dear Lord—I have to run to the finish?* Sweat is pouring off me. My legs are no longer bendable, I'm certain. In my mind I look like someone with stick legs trying to run down the hallway, but I make it to the mat, turn to my left and drop down against the wall.

I didn't remember until I viewed a video of my finish the next day that my teammates Ariel and Brian had greeted me with a handshake, a hug, and a bottle of water. I had no memory of it until I saw it on tape. I had seen myself crossing the mat on news video from the Strat climb, but this is different. Everyone's finish from this climb was taped. It's terrific.

We are allowed to walk around for a bit, so I soak in incredible views from the ninetieth floor for maybe ten minutes or so before we are directed downstairs to a lower floor. There organizers have prepared one of the nicest post-race layouts ever with lots of food and beverages and some swag and photo areas. Karen and I both thought it odd they were serving baked potatoes until we saw signs saying the little foil-wrapped bundles were breakfast burritos. I'm thrilled to see brewed decaf. I warn a couple of first timers not to get used to treatment like this. This is an especially nice after-party; most climbs do not put on a spread like we have here today.

There is a large paper banner on the wall for us to sign. Mark draws a WCL logo in the center. I see Jeannie writing a message on the banner, and then she also writes one amidst dozens on the wall, so I put a message there as well. I add Ariana's name after mine because I want her name to be there, too. Mariners Church always had us write our names on the floors or walls of new buildings, so writing my name on the wall here means a lot to me.

I chat with several first-time climbers and a couple of climbers I have not met previously, including the winner, forty-five year old Tim Donahue who scaled the Tower in 11:38. Tim was seventh in the 2015 Empire State Building Run-Up. Sproule Love, who beat Tim at the ESBRU, is second today with 11:58. Mark, who is having knee issues from years of running, still finishes in 15:18, twenty-sixth overall.

Gorgeous Stephanie Hucko from Florida is fastest overall female with 13:57. Stephanie was also fastest overall female at the U.S. Championships at the Stratosphere in March.

I ended up seventh in my AG with 22:58, behind Lisa (17:42), Karen Geninatti (18:27), Jeannie (20:52), and four other lovely fifty-five to fifty-nine-year-old ladies. Lisa is sixth overall female, Madeleine is eighth with 18:22, and Karen is ninth. Today's climb organized participants into five-year age groups, which is fairer to climbers at the upper ends of their age groups. Three of the top ten finishers in both the male and female categories are between the ages of fifty and sixty. Not too shabby.

Lisa, Madeleine, and I try to do a second climb, but we aren't allowed. We know it's a long shot, but we ask anyway. Several of us go back and climb our fifty-story, 804-step hotel stairwell afterward since we're still amped up.

Climb organizers did an amazing job, raising over half a million dollars to build a high-tech house for a veteran of the war in Afghanistan. Retired Army Sgt. Bryan Dilberian lost both legs and his left arm in combat. As a beneficiary of the climb, he felt compelled to participate and scaled the building in 1:08:57 with the help of prosthetics.

If he can do it, so can you.

CHAPTER TWENTY

Future Steps

I went from fat to fit in a little over two years by making significant changes in my diet and by exercising daily, usually walking. None of these changes would have taken place if I hadn't signed up to do my first stair climb. Each time I said yes to an opportunity, I reaped multiple benefits. In this book, I use the word *no* ten times as much as the word *yes*. Just like Jim Carrey in the movie *Yes Man*, saying yes at inappropriate times can create big problems, but when it comes to getting active and staying fit and healthy, the "yes" word may be your key to fitness.

Most of my improvement took place over a nine-month period in 2010, thanks to simply exercising more and eating less. I don't exercise hard every day, but I do something every single day, even if I just take the dogs for a nice brisk walk. The more time I spend being active, the less time I have to think about food and or indulge in eating.

Not everyone has access to stairs where they can work out. In my little hometown of Vinco, there are no public stairwells, and I doubt there's a building higher than three stories. If I still lived there, I would have to drive ten miles to find the nearest tall building or parking structure. Stair climbing is a wonderful way to improve fitness, but if you can't climb, walk. If walking is too boring, run. If running is too hard on you, swim. If you don't have access to a pool, bike. If you don't have a bike, buy or borrow one.

Whatever you do, move—and keep moving as much as possible. There's yoga, Pilates, barre, Zumba, tennis, bowling, skiing, surfing, paddleboarding. If you don't mind the gym, go to the gym. Find an exercise buddy—he or she will help keep you accountable. If having no legs or being eighty years old doesn't stop a person from climbing tall buildings, what's your excuse for not getting out there and being active?

Set goals. Find someone to inspire you. My dentist had always wanted to run a marathon, so he began training and ran his first marathon, the LA Marathon, when he turned fifty. Margarita Stocker ran her first marathon at age seventy.

In 2011 I was one of the top sixty women climbers in the world, and in 2014 I was ranked the number sixteen female climber in the U.S. I finished the 2015 season at number forty-six. I have not improved my time in every race. I still struggle every single day with hunger and keeping my weight down. I often suffer with self-esteem issues and feeling that I am not "good enough." Some days I find myself nearly crippled by self-doubt and anxiety. My experiences with stair climbing help me overcome these issues when they arise. I ask myself, *How much worse than climbing Willis could this particular challenge or obstacle be? If I can climb the country's tallest buildings and climb them well, what* can't *I accomplish?*

For much of my life I was angry with God for not giving me a loving, nurturing family. If he can do anything, why couldn't he have arranged things so that I had better parents, a more normal childhood, one that enabled me to be the person God created me to be? Later I accepted the fact that my parents had done the best they could, and God used my traumatic past to bring me into a loving relationship with him. Only recently I realized that my childhood was truly a gift. I don't need lots of money or material possessions to be happy. I really do enjoy life's simple pleasures: being in good health, having good friends, and living in a safe and peaceful environment.

I encourage you to make the most of what you have. Find something you like doing, give it your best effort, and enjoy every facet of it: the exercise, the experience, and those involved in it with you. Find a hero and emulate him or her. My stair climbing family encourages me every single day in one way or another. If you don't become a member of our extended step-family, I hope you'll find a community of your own where you will be fit and thrive.

If you do give tower running a try, I hope to see you some climb soon. If I can do it, you can, too.

Jeff Dinkin

When I met Jeff at my first climb in 2008, he was covered with road rash (brush burns) from a cycling accident earlier in the week and had one arm in a sling. I thought he was crazy to be racing up a tall building. Jeff's distinctive personality has earned him the nickname "Stair Climb Lunatic." He's known for bouncing straight up in the air while awaiting race starts, both to warm up and to help calm his nerves. Candid photos taken at climbs show Jeff seemingly suspended a foot above the ground.

He found out about competitive climbing when a cycling buddy posted a video of his 2006 U.S. Bank Climb on YouTube. Once Jeff got into the sport, he realized there were "tons of climbs" around the country and it was kind of a big thing. Jeff has completed nearly sixty climbs to date. His favorite is the Stratosphere in Las Vegas because it's such a unique structure with long flights and a very open feel. He's not as fond of Seattle's Big Climb due to the large number of competitors and says he climbed horribly in that building in three attempts.

Jeff is a fierce competitor who pushes himself to be faster and better each year. He climbs because he loves the people he meets in the sport. Jeff says stair climbers are "a profoundly kind group of like-minded people who all seem to enjoy, and even attribute some of their own personal success to, their ability to conquer tall buildings. It's very empowering, as those who do it understand." He also loves trail racing and used to race bicycles, but has replaced that with racing stairs, which is safer, and "has much nicer competitors."

For most of 2010 and part of 2011, a rather serious back injury impeded Jeff's ability to be active in any capacity, requiring him to spend a lot of time in bed. He bounced back from that difficult time in late 2011 and started doing better than ever before in races in 2012, with even further improvement in 2013 and 2014. He is still progressing and improving.

Jeff's training consists of a mix of cycling, trail running, and stair practice. Being in the Los Angeles area, outdoor training is possible year round. He says he is constantly learning about new places to train, which keeps training enjoyable. He trains an average of eight to ten hours a week. "It's a commitment, but it's not an outrageous amount of time. It's doable when you want it."

Jeff has a special relationship with most of his climbing friends. He says, "Yes, we actually refer to them as our 'step-family' (a pun on steps, or stairs). We are very close and enjoy each other very much. We often train together, have meals together, and encourage each other. It's an amazingly tight community of great people that I feel fortunate to be a part of."

He is inspired by a lot of people, not necessarily anyone famous, or even someone who has done something seemingly impossible. He is more inspired by people who step outside their comfort zone and find a way to overcome their own personal challenges, whatever they may be. He says those who inspire him are "literally too many to name.

"I'm inspired by each and every person who accepts the challenge to climb a building and get to the top. It's a very empowering feeling, and you can see the sense of accomplishment when they do it. Having been involved in this sport for a long time, it never gets easier, but it's always rewarding, and seeing others share in that feeling is inspiring in itself."

Jeff doesn't listen to music while training or racing. "I don't knock people who do, but it doesn't work for me."

Jeff's advice to aspiring stair climbers is: "Strive to be your best self and be passionate about what you love and enjoy; put your heart into it. Even when things aren't fun or easy, cultivating a mind-set of joy makes the difficult times go by easier and quicker."

PJ Glassey

I don't know when I first met the very fit PJ Glassey, owner of X Gyms in Seattle, but it was probably at the 2008 U.S. Bank Climb. He looks very serious, but he has a silly sense of humor and is a prolific health and fitness blogger. PJ, who turns fifty in 2016, did his first climb, the Big Climb in Seattle, in 2006 and has completed well over fifty climbs since. He did his first climb out of curiosity, before meeting Jeff Dinkin, who told him there were climbs all around the country.

"Jeff invited me to Sears, so I went, stayed with Jesse Berg, met Mark T., and based on getting to know them and other awesome people, I was hooked!"

Jesse Berg has inspired PJ to excel. Jesse "has the most amazing attitude, phenomenal talent, and is one of the most humble people I have ever known," PJ says.

PJ's least favorite climb is Chicago's Sears Tower, which is "way too long." His favorite climb, like Jeff's, is the Stratosphere in Vegas. It has an "awesome stairwell and a great turnout of stair-climbing buds."

PJ has had to overcome issues with pronation (the foot rolling inward during walks and runs) and resulting gait issues that prevent him from doing impact sports. He climbs "mostly because of the awesome people in the sport, but also for proof that my X Gym exercise methods work." (The X Gym exercise system is based on two twenty-one-minute workouts per week). He trains on an incline trainer, Jacob's Ladder, and stairs. His only prerace ritual is prayer, and while he doesn't listen to music during climbing, he often uses a metronome for pacing.

PJ says stair climbing is "the safest sport yet also the most challenging because it stretches you in many ways—especially in the areas of strength, endurance, and mental toughness. No other sport requires such high levels of all three of those categories at the same time."

To see a shirtless PJ and his six-pack abs and learn more about his fitness methods, go to pjfit.com, xgym.com, or stairsport.com.

Tommy Coleman

The fact that Tommy Coleman won his very first stair climb—the seventy-five-story U.S. Bank Climb in Los Angeles—and set a record there in 2013 speaks volumes about the way Tommy tackles life. Born in 1974, Tommy is a motorcycle mechanic, fashion accessories designer, and premed student. He likes to say he started climbing because he "had long looked for an extreme discipline that required immense suffering" and found it in tower running competitions. The U.S. Bank Tower Climb is his favorite because it's his hometown event, as well as his first. He likes climbs with fast competition; they motivate him to run hard.

He says he climbs to help complete his life with the essential physical fitness test/challenge component. "I also get excited when I think about cycling up mountains, running on uneven terrain, or swimming in the ocean when the surf is huge."

Tommy has only done about ten climbs. In 2013, he was diagnosed with a rare spinal disease known as syringomyelia—a neurologic-based malady that can cause myriad symptoms across many body systems. He is searching for another cause for his symptoms and hasn't trained for over a year. "I'm getting more anxious than ever to figure this thing out and get back up into the sky!" Tommy says.

He is inspired by "any speed demon, male or female. I tend to feel most connected to those who are invested in the analysis of the sporting life and how it relates to diet, injury, and disease."

When asked if he has a good luck charm, he said he makes his "own luck with a proper warm-up and a pole position start." He listens to Gangster rap or death metal while climbing, depending on his mood, and he admits that some of his training methods are "scary."

"Through stair sport and other athletic disciplines, I have procured valuable tools that I employ in everyday life. From high-level organization strategies to practices of sacrifice, I use what I have learned through training and racing to elevate my academic aptitude and proficiency in the workplace."

Check out Tommy's designs at www.tommytuckerjeans.com.

Lisa Zeigel

My step-sister Lisa is the program manager for the Fitness Center at the J. Paul Getty Center in Los Angeles. She began stair climbing when she worked as a program director for the South Pasadena San-Marino YMCA, which is affiliated with the Downtown-Ketchum Y.

"I kept getting bugged by colleagues to do the U.S. Bank Climb, so I finally said yes. I went to the practice climbs, and while we were doing them in the Wells Fargo building, 9/11 happened. I was certain the event would be canceled, but it wasn't. The climb took on a whole new meaning. In addition, I received a third-place age group medal on my first climb, so I was hooked! U.S. Bank was my first, and for the longest time I thought it was the only stair climb race in existence."

Lisa is currently ranked the number seventeen female in the world at the age of fifty-seven. While the U.S. Bank Climb is her favorite because it was her first, the Stratosphere is her least favorite. "I hate the stairwell, and I am not a fan of Vegas."

Lisa says, "Stair climbing keeps me out of trouble—somewhat. Really, it keeps me in great shape; I can spend less time doing stairs with better results than running or other cardio for longer duration. It keeps me mentally focused, and it probably keeps me young! I've been through eating disorders and alcohol addiction; I got in lots of trouble as a punk rocker in my early twenties. Before I started stair climbing, I was just getting over the worst of fibromyalgia, which was really debilitating for me in the mid to late nineties. Through diet and stress management, I was able to bring the symptoms down to minimal. Lately I have been battling sleep issues, but that's slowly getting better."

Lisa says she trains on stairs as much as possible and also sometimes uses stair machines. "I love training on the Manhattan Beach sand dunes," she says. "Strength training for total body balance is essential for me." Lisa's favorite step-siblings are, "to name a few, you, Jane; Jeannie, Madeleine, Jeff, Stan and Kathleen, David Garcia, Maria Martinez and Javier Santiago, Scott Stanley, Terryl DeBruin and Gary Baker. I could go on. Not only are they friends in stair climbing, but I have done things outside of the sport with many of them; they have put me up in their homes and driven me around when I visit from out of town. I feel like they would do almost anything for me—as I would for them. I truly feel like they are family. It's a great feeling to have that in my life."

Stair climbing "unexpectedly became more than a hobby" for Lisa, a vegan. Once she saw that she was "ranked," it made her want to train harder and do more climbs. "The best thing of all is that it has given me an added incentive to travel; I've been to places I might not have gone to without participating in stair-climbing races: Mexico City, Chicago, New York, Dallas, Seattle. I always meet new people and have exciting adventures that enrich my life in general. I plan to keep stair climbing into my seventies, eighties, and beyond. It would be cool to be in my nineties and still climb. It keeps me young in mind and body, and the social aspect can't be beat. I hope your readers get just as inspired by the sport!"

Karen Geninatti

Fifty-eight-year-old personal trainer Karen Geninatti did her first climb way back in 1980 at the Springfield Hilton and has done well over fifty climbs since then. She's not sure how many—she's lost count. She is tiny in stature but huge in enthusiasm in anything she tackles. Karen is currently ranked the twenty-fifth best female climber in the world.

"Thirty years ago I competed in running events, marathons, half marathons, and 5ks. I then competed in bodybuilding on the national level for twelve years. I was looking for a new way to challenge myself, and I certainly found it in tower running."

Karen loves all the climbs, but she says the U.S. Bank Climb is a favorite. "I love the camaraderie, the atmosphere, and the all-day party. I get to see so many climbing friends. It is nice that the hotel is so close by, and it's a very well-run event." At the bottom of her list is the Springfield Hilton. "It's funny because I have a team of 131 who competes in it. But it's my home turf, and it's so hard to be on top of my game when I have my team to look after. I would rather just be there for my team."

Karen trains six days a week, approximately three hours a day. She prays while waiting in the starting line. When asked if she has a special relationship with any of her step-siblings, she said, "Definitely." She is inspired by: "Mark Block and many others: David Hanley, Madeleine Ronk, Nelson Quong, Oz Osborn, Syd Arak, Bob Toews, Jason Larson, Josh Duncan, Eric Lenenger, Kristin Frey, Tommy Coleman, Alex Workman, Veronica Stocker, Cindy Harris, Jeff Dinkin. Really, our whole stair-climbing family."

Karen says *anyone* can do this. "I have seen people climb stairs on crutches, with one leg, on oxygen, and most inspiring, Mark Block, who climbs stairs after being paralyzed twice in his life and told he would never move again, let alone walk."

The only place you can find Karen standing still is at www.kareng online.com.

Jeannie Rasmussen

I met Jeannie at her first climb, the 2010 AON Climb in Los Angeles. She met my brother Mark in 1990 through her job as print buyer/traffic manager for Trader Joe's in their corporate office. She and Mark were born less than a month apart in 1959. "Mark and I have had a working relationship and friendship for the last twenty-six years. He got me into stair climbing—I don't know whether to thank him or hate him. Just kidding!"

Jeannie has completed about twenty climbs, and her favorite is the Cystic Fibrosis Climb in Los Angeles because she likes the metal steps. She doesn't like AON's concrete steps and left-hand turns.

When Jeannie was twenty-one, she was in a motorcycle accident that broke her pelvis and cracked her helmet. "I thank God I was wearing one!" she says. "I had a recovery period of about eight weeks. I told myself to never take for granted the gift of movement." She has issues with her left knee and periodic right hamstring issues. Her mother has type 2 diabetes, and it runs in her family. "I've always included exercise and eating well as a part of my life to avoid contracting type 2 diabetes myself."

Jeannie trains in the buildings where the stair races are being held whenever she can. She trains to mostly seventies rock music. "I don't race with music, though; I want to hear myself breathe. I train at least three times a week in my gym, running, using the stair-climbing machine and/or the elliptical trainer (I do some sort of cardio for half an hour), weights for another half hour, conclude with sit ups, then stretch for ten minutes." She climbs for the "physical challenge, competition, and West Coast Labels team support" and is a medal-winning 5k runner who prays before competitions.

She is inspired by her twin sister and all of her step-siblings. "I especially admire Madeleine Ronk for her strength while battling breast cancer. She continues to train with such amazing spirit. She gives it her all no matter how difficult it may be, and she's always smiling! Since I started stair climbing and racing with the West Coast Labels team, I've had such a wonderful time being part of a fantastic group of athletes. My 5k racing has also improved by adding stair climbing and racing to my training skill set. In my fifty to fifty-four and fifty-five to fifty-nine age groups, I've enjoyed medaling in numerous 5k events as a result of stair climbing."

Johnny Ravello

Johnny "Johnny Rocket" Ravello won his first ever climb, the 2010 U.S. Bank Climb in Los Angeles, at the age of nineteen. "I was bored with my cardio workout [cycling]. The local gym I am a member of organizes the YMCA Climb for LA every year, so I decided to try it." Johnny climbs for fun and to stay in shape, and he also participates in baseball, hockey, and hiking. He hikes a lot and goes to the gym regularly to train.

When asked who inspires him, Johnny said, "All my friends and family inspire me in different ways, I suppose. But if you're asking about athletes I admire, Tommy Caldwell, Alex Honnold, and Ueli Steck are three."

Johnny says, "Here's the deal. I started stair climbing for fun. Not because I was in poor health and had to choose an activity to live a healthy lifestyle. Not because I had an illness or injury that forced me to change my way of living. I started stair climbing just for the fun of it. I like to challenge myself physically. It's a good feeling when you do that, and I am glad I chose stair climbing because not only did I find something fun and rewarding, but I also met and befriended genuinely nice people, too. My story isn't as inspiring as others in the WCL crew, but I don't think you need an inspirational story to get motivated to do these kinds of things. You either love being active and challenging yourself or you don't."

I once encountered Johnny in the elevator at practice (going down, of course), and he was wearing a fifty-pound vest. He was completely drenched in sweat and was wearing the extra weight to improve his strength and stamina.

He really does love a challenge.

George Burnham

Retired carpenter and electrician George Burnham is a legend among climbers. Born in 1942, George did his first climb in Phoenix in 1996 at the age of fifty-four. It was a two-hour climb to raise money for cystic fibrosis. He climbed the building eleven times, and he did it sixteen times the year after. The 2016 Scale the Strat Climb will be his 174th lifetime climb. The Stratosphere is one of George's favorites, along with the Benington, Vermont, Monument Climb.

George says, "Climbing gives me something to do. I like the exercise, and the different charities are good causes." He was never really athletic but used to cycle. George has had asthma since 1966. "I've had arthroscopic knee surgery, and I had a heart bypass on October 30, 2012. I did my first two climbs after that on the same weekend in January 2013—one in Dallas, the other in Portland."

George competes so often that he doesn't need to train, but he does the stairs in the city park in Phoenix. "There are twenty-one steps. I do it ten to thirteen times whenever I can," he says.

"People tell me they can't do what I do, and I tell them they can. I always wear my team jersey and my medal (when I get one) on the flight after a climb. I was on my way to Fort Worth from a climb for the National Fallen Firefighters Association, and the guy in the seat next to me asked me about my jersey. When I told him what I did, he was so impressed that he said he wanted to sponsor my next climb (the CF climb in Fort Worth) and gave me two one hundred dollar bills. He gave me a ride to Fort Worth in his expensive sports car; we got stuck in the snow and had to have the car towed. The climb was cancelled due to the bad weather, so I used the money to fund the climb I did after that one."

Wayne Hunkins

Wayne—aka Sam—Hunkins is an attorney in the process of retiring. He made his first climb at the Empire State Building in 2013 at the age of seventy-seven. He's done about seventeen climbs to date.

Wayne said he had a problem getting up from the floor. "I have a couple of friends my age who are so feeble they have trouble getting in and out of a car. I decided I was just plain not going there." He enjoys climbing because "it is the only heavy cardio that does not seem to have some serious negative consequence for me." Wayne, who smoked for five years, is inspired by his mother, who was active beyond the age of one hundred.

Wayne trains like me, in parking structures. He goes up the stairway and down the elevator. "They're usually open 24/7. I do the occasional tall building as well as the Baldwin Hills Overlook. A typical morning climb would be about a hundred floors. I've found that a ten-to-twelve-floor climb forty-five minutes before competitions works wonders."

Wayne says, "Use it or lose it. Medical studies show that most elderly persons can improve their mobility and function substantially by simple regular exercise. I am serious about climbing many of the world's tallest buildings at eighty, thus my website URL. As I get closer to ninety, I plan to try out the motivational speaker circuit."

Get the latest on Wayne at stairclimb-at-80.com.

Stan Schwarz

The first time I saw Stan was memorable: He passed me on all fours in the AON stairwell at his first climb in 2009. He was wearing running shorts, and his many tattoos were visible. I teased him afterward that he climbed like Spiderman. Stan, a computer systems administrator, is in the extremely competitive 50–59 AG category so he seldom medals, but he always gives a climb everything he's got. He has at least thirty climbs under his belt.

"Susan Opas was the one who first told me how to find stair events, so she's the reason I got so involved in this crazy sport. I thought it would be an interesting physical challenge, and I wanted to be able to stand on the roof of the AON building," Stan explains. When I asked him why he continues to climb, he said, "It's still an interesting physical challenge. And I've got a whole social circle out of doing this crazy sport. It's fun to visit and see everyone."

Stan's favorite climb is the San Diego Towerthon. "Traditionally I do better at competitions that are longer, as opposed to fast sprints." That's one reason the ALA San Diego Climb is his least favorite. "At thirty-four stories, the building is just too short."

He trains by "riding my bike, doing practice climbs downtown when I can, and doing stairs at Millikan Library at Caltech. I ride my bike a lot. I've been a big cyclist since 1973." He got a great workout by climbing the Wilshire-Figueroa building 101 times over the course of a year in 2013.

Stan is our numbers guy. "I started counting steps in 2012 when I was trying to work out the most efficient step patterns to take the minimum number of steps. The whole idea was to eliminate taking extra steps on the landings while turning. I figured that taking an extra step costs a half second or so, and multiplying that by two landings per floor and fifty to seventy-five floors adds up to some time. So I figured out a pattern that worked on the AON building stairs: Put a single foot on the landing, pivot, and start each flight left foot first. The pattern repeats, with no wasted steps. I began doing that in practice, and I started noticing that, while it was efficient, my left leg seemed to be working harder than the right. I paid attention and noticed that the flights were eleven steps each. That meant doing three doubles with the left leg and two doubles and a single on the right. So the left leg was working 20 percent harder than the right. When I alternated putting the single step at the beginning or the end of each eleven-step flight, it alternated which leg worked harder. So now I do this change every five floors to even out the load on the legs.

"After I started thinking about stepping patterns, I started paying more attention to the step configurations, and I started wondering if the published step counts they had for the buildings were right. I saw that Kevin Crossman had made a detailed chart for the building he works and trains in, so I decided to make one for the AON building. I figured this would help to work out the best step patterns for the different sections of the staircase, and it also would help work out split times for pacing. So I walked up slowly on one of the practice nights, taking detailed notes. When I made up the chart, I found that the published count of 1,377 was wrong. A later review found a couple of small errors in my chart, but that's the story of how I started making the stair charts."

Check out Stan's stats at www.1134.org.

Kourtney Dexter

I've only done a couple of climbs with Kourtney, who is all smiles and positive energy. Her first climb was the Columbia Tower in Seattle. "PJ asked me to race the Columbia Tower in 2008 and I won, so he encouraged me to do more. Thanks, Peej! PJ is my brother from another stepmother, that's for sure. He got me into climbing, encouraged my training, and believed in me when I doubted myself. He teaches me something new with every conversation. Nelson is my step-bestie and the male version of me. Roxanne (Sanchez) kills it at life—she totally inspires me."

Of the more than two dozen climbs Kourtney has completed, the Benningon Monument in Vermont is her favorite. It's a "short, sweet sprint in a rad building!" she says. On the other hand, the Presidential Towers Climb in Chicago is four buildings with a sprint between each one and is "so not up my alley."

She is "retired" now, but she climbed to raise funds for various charities "and, of course, to overcome self-imposed limitations." She is now into racewalking. When asked how she trains, she said she does "anything but climb stairs. Or run. Or use the elliptical."

At the tender age of thirty-six, Kourtney has already dealt with a "broken back, arthritis in my hips, and a torn meniscus, rotator cuff, and TFL (tensor fasciae latae)."

For workouts, Kourtney listens to hip-hop or audiobooks; for competitions, it's classic slow rock.

Kourtney's philosophy? "Don't take it so seriously. Moderation is healthy. No excuses or big talk. Just go out and do your thing!"

Veronica Stocker

Pretty blonde Veronica Stoker, also known as "V" or "Vero," is stair climbing's glamour girl. But don't get in this beauty's way in the stairwell—she'll blow your doors off. Veronica has been competing since she climbed the U.S. Bank Tower in 2004 at the age of thirty-four, and she's lost count of the number of buildings she's conquered since. Veronica is currently ranked the number-six female in the world. She finished the 2015 season at number two in the country behind another lovely blonde, Stephanie Hucko (towerrunningusa.com currently tracks over twenty thousand females in the U.S.).

A Spanish interpreter by day, forty-seven-year-old Veronica got involved in stair climbing when her boyfriend at the time "encouraged me to sign up because I was always training on the stair-climbing machine at the gym." She stuck with it for "fitness, the challenge, the feeling of accomplishment, and the charity organizations." Veronica trains on stairs and hill repeats, rides a spin bike, uses weights, and runs. She is a medal-winning runner as well.

The U.S. Bank Climb is her favorite because it was her first. The Stratosphere is her least favorite: "It always takes me a couple of weeks to recover from that race. I think it's because the air is so dry in Las Vegas or something. I am coughing and sneezing for days after that event."

When asked about her step-siblings, Veronica said, "I consider a few to be some of my closest friends. They understand me. My friends who are not athletes cannot fully relate to what I do or appreciate why I devote so much time, effort, and money to this sport. My step-siblings totally get it! Many people in my life—some who are no longer with me—inspire me. I also inspire myself, because my road has been a long one. I was not always an athlete, far from it, and only I know how much blood, sweat, and tears it took to get to the point where I am today. I am motivated by the idea of setting a good example for my son as well." Veronica's teenage son is a top contender in his AG, her mother, Margarita, is a top climber in the seventy and over AG, and her father has climbed also.

Veronica has a "certain necklace" that she wears every race. She says, "I always pray before a race, and I remember all those who have inspired me; I also focus my thoughts on the people I dedicate my runs to. I never listen to music during a race or during my workouts and trainings. The motivation has to come from within. Music is an artificial motivator—one learns to depend on it. I don't want to depend on anything but my own willpower. It' s just a personal preference; it's what works for me."

Veronica's philosophy? "Don't live vicariously through others. If you have a passion or an interest, just go for it. It's great to admire other people for what they do or for what they have achieved, but be your own hero as well."

Michael "Mike" Caviston

How fit do you have to be when your job description is "promoting physical fitness in the military"? Take one look at fifty-five-year-old Mike Caviston, and you know immediately.

Mike's first climb was the 2010 U.S. Bank Climb, and he's done at least forty climbs since.

Mike was looking for a new challenge. "I used to specialize in one sport, rowing, but decided it was time to diversify. Now I fit stair climbs into a busy competition schedule that includes lots of road and trail runs and the odd triathlon, snowshoe, kayak, or rowing (erg) races." He trains by doing "a variety of things: running (lots of hills), rowing (C2 erg), stair climbs, lots of cycling (I don't own a car), and some weight lifting. I train 365 days a year, and there are no 'easy' days—just hard in different ways."

If he listens to music when he works out, he says, "It's a lot of genres, but lots of oldies and classic rock."

Mike is a big "calories in, calories out" kind of guy who eats what he wants, within reason, and then burns it all off. Mike likes to eat and likes to read. He also "likes to eat while reading."

When I asked Mike about his favorite climb, he said, "I liked Scale the Strat a lot when it was a two-day event. Now I'm not sure which is my favorite. I like that most climbs are unique and hard to compare." He's not crazy about Willis Tower "only because I've never raced well there. It is actually a great climb."

When I asked him why he climbs, Mike responded, "Because it's there. Or, if you have to ask, you wouldn't understand. As my knees get older and complain more, climbing is less stressful than other sports. I'm asthmatic, but I manage it pretty well."

His prerace ritual is to "get up early, have a Cliff bar and a cup of coffee, visualize the race, and get a good warm-up."

As for his step-family, Mike says, "They are all a great bunch of people who I don't see much between races, but on race day we pick right up like we've known each other forever."

He is inspired by "explorers, those who challenged the unknown, especially the polar regions. Trekking across Antarctica for months with no chance of rescue if you fail puts climbing a building for ten minutes into perspective. Same with stories of those who were lost at sea, were POWS, etc."

Not only does Mike not own a car, but he says, "I don't use Facebook and barely comprehend the Internet or cell phones, so don't bother calling either."

Mike's advice: "Climbing is a good metaphor for all of life's challenges and problems. Even if you're going to climb the tallest building in the world, just take it one step at a time and don't stop till you reach the top. Okay, I literally climb two stairs at a time, but it is still one step . . ."

Madeleine Fontillas Ronk

Forty-eight-year-old Madeleine Ronk is a stair-climbing powerhouse who has managed to get her entire family—her husband, son, and three daughters—involved in the sport since her first climb at the U.S. Bank Tower in 2004. She has more than sixty climbs under her belt and is currently the number fourteen female climber in the world.

Madeleine used to work in a thirty-story building in downtown Los Angeles. "After the events of September 11, 2001, a coworker and I decided to practice descending the stairs so we could save our own lives in the event of an earthquake, fire, or terrorist attack. We would race down the stairs, and it took only minutes. We decided to make it a lunchtime workout and added going up the stairs, too. It was a great workout and the pounds from the birth of my second child just melted off. In 2004 we saw signs for a stair climb being held at the U.S. Bank Tower two blocks from our office. We signed up, and that was the start of my competitive tower-running madness."

Madeleine is one of the fortunate few who were chosen to do "La Verticale de la Tour Eiffel," the Eiffel Tower Climb, and it's her favorite. "It's an exclusive, exciting, and prestigious climb in the most well-known and iconic structure in the world. What better way to see and experience Paris than from the internal belly of the Eiffel Tower?" She loves the ESBRU, but admits that she hates "how grueling it is with its steep, tall steps, the extra long flights, landings in between flights, and my inability to run that race in a decent time. One day I'll conquer that building, but I'll have to train like a beast to do it."

A recent breast cancer survivor, Madeleine is a carrier of the BRCA1 gene mutation. "Although I opted out of chemotherapy, I've had a bilateral mastectomy, had my lymph nodes removed, and have been in the 'reconstruction zone' for two years due to several infections and implant failures. Needless to say, my pectoral strength is compromised. I've endured ten surgeries/hospitalizations during the past two years, but I've tried to schedule my surgeries around my race schedule—or raced against the advisement of my doctors. The cancer medications and antibiotics have caused joint and ligament issues in my shoulders and knees, so I often have to work through pain when I train and race. As long as I can still climb, however fast or slow, I will not quit because it's an activity that I love and am passionate about. My husband and children are my biggest inspirations and motivators. I try to stay fit and healthy for them so I can be the best mom and wife I can be."

She climbs building stairwells to train at every opportunity and also climbs the many public outdoor stairways in her neighborhood. Madeleine likes pop songs with driving messages in the lyrics. "Run Away Baby" by Bruno Mars and "The Final Bell" from the movie soundtrack from *Rocky* are a few of her favorites. She also likes Demi Lovato, "Killing in the Name Of" by Rage Against the Machine and "Levitate" by Hodouken! She has only one prerace ritual: "Right before I'm told 'Go!' at the start, I always make the Sign of the Cross three times; I ask God to help me do my best and keep me safe."

Madeleine loves her step-family. "Each one of them has offered me motivation, inspiration, and support in my sport and life in general. Even step-siblings I know only through social media are special friends I'm privileged to know."

Madeleine offers these words of wisdom: "No matter what the obstacle is before you in life, keep climbing, keep stepping—crawl if you must, but just keep aiming toward the finish line."

Learn more about this courageous lady at www.beachbody.com/MadSteppingStrong or find her on Instagram @mfontillasronk.

Alberto Lopez

I first met Alberto, aka "AO" or "Bert," in the stairwell at my first Towerthon in San Diego. He's done about twenty climbs and started when he was twenty-nine years old in 2009.

A former educator, Alberto says his students were his inspiration. "We can see the tallest building west of the Mississippi (U.S. Bank Tower in Los Angeles) from the school playground. At the time the kids were in awe of Spiderman. So I told them I could climb as Spiderman did. And my stair-climbing life began."

The AON building in LA is his favorite climb "because of the difficulty of the stairs," and he also likes the San Diego Towerthon for "mentally pushing your body further than you ever have." He says seeing the same smiling faces brings him joy.

"Stair climbing has been my physical therapy for my knees. My doctor told me to do lunges and squats to allow the muscles to get stronger. Stair climbing does that for me. I chose to not have a car. Because of that, I cycle everywhere. I also do crossfit, swim, track endurance, and stairs in the building where I live. There are only two floors, but that happens to work for me. I am also a volunteer pacer for a local running group, A Runners Circle."

When asked if he has a special relationship with any of his stepsiblings, Alberto's response was, "All of them! I am always at a happy place with every single one of them. Madeleine encouraged me to be part of the team (WCL). Jeff Dinkin has always pushed me to be better and quicker in the stairs. Nandor has spiritual conversations with me. I get what I need from all without asking. They just give, and I hope

I can do the same for them. It's a positive, competitive, encouraging, helpful group."

Alberto says he's inspired by anyone he comes in contact with. "For good or bad, you can always internalize it and make it positive. We get to live this one life, and we should be inspired by all."

Marisol Ronk

I typically refer to soon-to-be fifteen-year-old Marisol Ronk as "my little nemesis." Since our first climb together when she knocked me out of the top ten, we have almost always finished within a few seconds of one another. I usually nose her out in the taller buildings; she bests me in the shorter ones. Her first climb was the U.S. Bank in 2010 when she was nine, and she's completed over thirty climbs.

She started because her mom, Madeleine, is one of the top climbers in the world. Marisol is currently ranked number sixteen in her AG. She climbs because it's fun and adds, "I climb for those who can't." Her favorite climb is the ALA San Diego because "it's short, a sprint." Her least favorite climb is the Sears/Willis because "it's long, and the steps are tall." She trains by doing triathlons—she's done three—and she does the practice climbs when she can. She also is active in gymnastics and scuba diving, and she took dance for ten years.

She is closest to her step-siblings Veronica and Matias, Veronica's son. Marisol listens to her current favorite songs during competitions. "I put them in order, and I make sure the last one is upbeat and fast."

Marisol says stair climbing is "kind of a unique sport, and it's good exercise. It's a way to support charities, and it's fun, too."

Imelda Briseno de Altamirano

It's not always easy communicating with foreign climbers, but Imelda Briseno has a smile that breaks through any language barrier. When her smile doesn't work, she just gives you a giant hug. The homemaker from Guadalajara, Jalisco, Mexico, did her first climb in 2010 at the Latin Tower in Mexico City. She has completed about thirty climbs since in the United States and Mexico, and she wears her titanium PHITEN necklace for each climb.

She started stair climbing because her husband loved it. She says, "It is a great challenge and extraordinary exercise. I love yoga and work out a little at the gym. I also like running, but I have a lot of injuries. Sometimes my hip hurts a little or my ankles swell a bit. My husband Luis trains me. On Monday, Wednesday, and Friday, I do about 150 floors, and on Tuesdays and Thursdays, I do a hundred floors for an easy workout." This comes from a woman born in 1954.

The entire group of climbers inspires Imelda, but she has special relationships with several step-siblings: Madeleine, Lisa, Steve, Nelson, Mark, Leland, Harish, PJ, Beverly, and yours truly.

"I have to train a lot and be very careful [not to gain weight] because every extra kilo means more of a load to carry up the stairs. I'm very happy climbing stairs," says Imelda, who is currently ranked second in her AG for the 2015 season in the U.S. rankings.

Cindy Levine

Cindy is a proud stay-at-home mom and freelance photographer who completed her first climb at the 2012 Towerthon. She took second place in her 40–49 AG, has done about twenty climbs since, and is currently ranked the number fifty female climber in the world.

"In 2011 I ran a half marathon and a marathon on two consecutive days, and as a result, I tore my medial meniscus on my right knee. So I did some research on low-impact sports for knees, and stair climbing came up. I've had knee and spine problems since I was a child, but with stair climbing, those problems are less of an issue. I love to compete, but mainly I climb to get a great workout for my lungs, heart, legs, and glutes." Cindy also loves to play tennis and trains at the gym doing the stairmill, spinning classes, and other arm and leg workouts. She says, "Stair climbing is a total workout that improves health, physical appearance, gains friends, and at the same time benefits charity, so it is a win-win cause!" Cindy and I like much of the same workout music: Billy Idol, Selena Gomez, Katy Perry, Lady Gaga, Rhianna.

"The Stratosphere is my favorite climb because it has fewer turns and is very spacious inside the building. The spaciousness makes it cool in temperature. I also love Vegas! The U.S. Bank is my least favorite because it starts at noon, and the building gets hot. It also occurs on a Friday, which means my son and husband can never be there to support me since they are busy with school and work."

Step-sisters Lisa and Karen inspire forty-four-year-old Cindy. "I want to become better at this wonderful sport and become the oldest women ever to climb a tower when I'm one hundred years old!"

Cindy does a Bible study before each race to find the "right Scripture that will make me feel strong while racing." Here are three of Cindy's favorite prerace Scriptures:

My brothers and sisters, be very happy when you are tested in different ways. You know that such testing of your faith produces endurance. (James 1:2–3)

Don't be afraid little flock. Your Father is pleased to give you the Kingdom. (Luke 12:32)

Trust the Lord with all your heart, and do not rely on your own understanding. In all your ways acknowledge him and he will make your path smooth. (Proverbs 3:5–6)

Learn more about Cindy at www.CindyLevineAthlete.com.

Luis Cesar Altamirano

Luis has a degree in business administration and owns a real estate and construction company, but his heart is with the staircases of the many buildings he's climbed, having done over forty climbs since his first in Mexico DF in 2007. He says he climbs to stay sane, have a healthy body, and ensure a better quality of life.

"I started running road races in 1979, but what I like now is to climb stairs. Climbing inspires me to achieve my goals to improve my times. I want to set an example for my family—my wife Imelda and my children—and my friends, too. Running on the street damaged my knees slightly, but I always ran with good shoes and insoles for my feet. I climb stairs Monday to Saturday. On Monday, Wednesday, and Friday, I do 150 floors. I do reps of five stories or combinations five to fifteen floors four times. On Tuesday, Thursday, and Saturday, I do an easy climb: one hundred floors one step at a time. Sunday I rest. If time allows, I cycle on my road bike about 35 kilometers twice a week."

Luis doesn't like listening to music when competing or when training. "It distracts me from what I'm doing. I try to concentrate in the days before a race on what I have accomplished. I always wear a chain around my neck with a gold runner that Imelda gave me as a gift when I turned fifty. I have never removed it."

Luis says what motivates him and keeps him going is being an example to others. Luis, who was born in 1950, says he has run over four hundred competitions, including thirty-eight full marathons, over one hundred half marathons, two ultra marathons of 50 km each, and other 5k and 10k races. "For eleven years, I helped prepare a group of about fifty people to run marathons and half marathons. I never charged any money—it was always free. In 2009 I decided to dedicate my time strictly to climbing buildings. I've never had an injury climbing, so I recommend it 100 percent."

David Hanley

Forty-three-year-old David Hanley is a computer programmer and vegan athlete who is also sports director for the U.S. Stair Climbing Association. He's completed about fifty climbs since his first climb at AON Chicago in 2009.

He started climbing because he was getting heavier and progressively more out of shape. "I decided to try to run around the block, and I couldn't even make it halfway down the block. I lifted weights at the gym a bit and I was too embarrassed to run on the treadmill, but the Stairmaster seemed like something I could do. It was less awkward-looking and no one would be able to tell how I was doing. I did it for a while and made some good gains. Then someone mentioned Hustle Up the Hancock, and I did the Chicago races for a while. Next I signed up for the Empire State lottery and got in! That encouraged me to train a bit more seriously. I started to make friends among the step-sibs, and I was hooked!" He continues to climb "to stay in shape, to inspire others to a healthy and active lifestyle, and to promote a diet of more plant foods."

David loves the Scale the Strat and U.S. Bank Climbs "because of the spectacle involved in both. And the fact that they usually involve a vacation and hiking trip on my part." On the other hand, he doesn't like Chicago's Presidential Towers due to the "tiny ugly staircase, constant turns, and the fact that it's four sprints."

David, currently the number forty-seven male climber in the world, started tracking climbers points out of personal interest. "I was intrigued by the fact I had a world ranking, though because I was far from the top 100, I could rarely tell where I stood; it was hard to see what races counted or if there was a mistake that was costing me points. With races in the U.S. being much larger, I thought a system that ranked everyone who raced—not just the top fifteen or thirty—would be a good idea. So I designed a scoring system that ranked everyone who raced while largely paralleling the world system. As a computer programmer, I was able to create some software that automated much of the work. Often a race only takes ten minutes to enter, though it can be much more at times. I find the scoring system very gratifying, because most weeks I get an e-mail from individuals who are overjoyed to see they have a national ranking. They often tell me they will now be training and working out more to try to improve their standing, so I'm happy to be leading people toward fitness in some small way."

David explains, "The system works by assigning points to races based on how competitive they are. A 200-point race will award 200 points to the winner, one-fifth fewer to second place, and so on. A person's standing at any given point is computed by summing up their five best scores from the past year. Top climbers in the nation often end up at a thousand points or higher. We also award age groups, which lets people compete and strive for higher rankings even if they're not in the top overall scorers. I'm glad I started the U.S. scoring system; it's a major way I feel I'm giving back for how stair climbing has improved my own life!"

Check out David's rankings at towerrunningusa.com.

Kathleen Andrew Schwarz

Kathleen is a supervising children's social worker in the Los Angeles County Department of Children and Family Services. She is married to Stan Schwarz and did her first climb in February 2011, the San Diego Fight for Air Climb. It was "just thirty-one floors!" says Kathleen. She has done about twenty more climbs.

She did her first climb at the age of fifty-three "to see if I could finish one. Also, I was tired of just standing around waiting for Stan and watching everyone else participate. I am not a competitive racer, and unfortunately I don't practice or train enough for it to improve my fitness. And I actually don't like climbing very much. But it's fun to be able to say that I've climbed these different buildings, and it does give me a sense of accomplishment when I've finished. Also we meet so many great people through the sport, who we maintain contact with through social media and get to see at the races." Kathleen said the only obstacle she has had to overcome to climb a tall building was her "inferiority complex."

Kathleen likes the Stratosphere in Las Vegas. "Most people don't like it, but it's fun because it's in Las Vegas, people travel to the race from all over the country (and even outside the U.S.), and I like looking down inside the open stairwell!" Like many of her step-siblings, her least favorite is the Willis Tower. "It's the tallest building I've ever climbed. I thought I was going to die."

When I asked her about training for the climbs, she said, "I think about training: *I really should train*. Then I kind of just show up. Maybe that's why I'm so slow!"

I asked her about what she considers the best part of this sport. She said, "It's getting to meet different people and making good friends who end up feeling like a sort of extended family." She is inspired by her step-family, especially Madeleine Fontillas Ronk and "those who have dealt with weight issues, including my brother John Andrew, David Garcia, and you, Jane!"

Kathleen has "lucky underwear" that she's worn for every climb. She says, "They're black-and-white-striped with a metallic silver thread. I'm not actually sure that they're especially lucky, though." While climbing, she listens to "loud hard rock or something with a heavy beat. Some stuff I like is from System of a Down, KONGOS, 'Shipping Up to Boston' from Dropkick Murphys, and 'Normal Person' from Arcade Fire. I also like dance music, like 'Dance Apocolyptic' from Janelle Monae. And, of course, 'Let It Go' from *Frozen* works really great, too!"

When asked what she would tell anyone who might be interested in stair climbing, Kathleen replied, "Whenever people find out that I do stair climbing, the most common things I hear are 'You must be in really good shape,' and 'I could never do that.' Neither of those things is true. I used to work out a lot, and I was pretty fit. I hope someday to get back to that, but right now, my work and commuting schedule just haven't made that possible (yeah, I know that's an excuse!). So I'm here as proof that anyone who can climb a flight or two of stairs can do one of these races. I just take my time, and I get there eventually. Along the way you get to meet new people, make great friends, and have an excuse to travel to new places! And if you do have time to practice and train, stair climbing really can help you get in great shape and improve your health and fitness. But even if that's not your goal, you can still have fun and get a lot out of the sport."

Steve Stermer

Sure-footed senior software engineer Steve Stermer develops satellite simulators used in government space programs for Lockheed Martin. His first competitive steps were on February 22, 2009, at the Run the Republic Climb in Denver, Colorado. He has done well over forty climbs in the nine years since.

"I received an email to join a Lockheed Martin corporate team for the Denver climb. I thought, *How hard could it be? It's just stairs.* Ten floors into the race, I realized how hard it could be, and afterward I was committed to improving my time the following year. I also started looking for other races around the country to pursue right away. I was hooked."

Fifty-eight-year-old Steve, currently ranked the world's number fifty-five male climber, is another fan of Scale the Strat in Las Vegas. "I loved the original format of a two-day climb, where you had to qualify in the top fifty to race up a second time the next day. They've moved to a single day format, but I still enjoy the atmosphere, the views, and the unique stairwell it provides. It is also the U.S. Championship race, so it draws the best climbers from across the country and usually has some international elites as well. It is a great place to reunite with many friends in the climbing community."

His least favorite climb is Willis Tower. "I've done this race several times and always seem to do much worse than I should. The steps are taller than in most other buildings, and something about the race just crushes my spirit. Someday I hope to go back and finally do well there."

I asked Steve why he enjoys stair climbing. "I climb for the fitness aspect as well as the community of climbers I've come to know through this sport. I've made friends with athletes from all over the United States, as well as Germany, Mexico, Canada, Denmark, Austria, and other countries. The community is so encouraging and supportive, even though we compete intensely with each other. I've never encountered a sore loser or seen any attitude less than positive. We all rejoice with our step-siblings when they do well, and encourage them when they have an off day."

Steve lives in Colorado, where he is "fortunate to have high-elevation training opportunities everywhere I look. I hike 14,000 ft. peaks and various trails up local mountains. I also ride many of the area's mountain bike trails. But most of my training is done on the Manitou Incline, a repurposed scenic railroad bed that rises two thousand feet over a one-mile span. The 2,800 railroad crossties form a staircase that climbs straight up the side of a mountain, topping out at an 8,500 ft. elevation. Surrounded by magnificent natural beauty, it offers a heart-pounding workout that I try to do at least once every day, regardless of the weather. Climbing it in snow is actually my favorite time." (Hence the reason I mention Steve's sure-footedness. He runs back down the incline even in icy weather).

Steve has "made so many lasting friendships with my fellow climbers that I would have otherwise missed out on. We are a very tight-knit group that keeps in contact online and at every race we can make. I always look forward to seeing them all at various races around the country. I see so many fellow climbers who have faced potentially devastating issues in their life and yet have conquered them to continue competing. From brain injuries and paralysis to cancers and knee injuries, this group is the embodiment of dedication, perseverance, and triumph."

Steve tries to "find songs that have beats that are near the step pacing I need to reach my goal. Fast-paced music with a very strong beat keeps my feet moving."

Steve says, "The old adage of 'one step at a time' is nowhere more fitting that in stair climbing. When faced with a seemingly insurmountable obstacle, the only way to attack it is in very small increments. Stair climbing is the ultimate exercise in stepwise refinement: Break the problem down into manageable chunks and then get through each one. Always remember that the pain will end soon. Eventually you will overcome the beast and celebrate your victory. Then start thinking about how you can do it better, faster, and more efficiently next time. The competition is less with other climbers than with yourself. Always strive to do better each time. Ultimately, the only one you need to beat is you."

Leland Jay

Leland Jay writes music and has done a couple of tongue-in-cheek rap songs about stair climbing, so Jeff Dinkin calls him "LL Stair J." Forty-seven-year-old Leland is a manufactured home dealer and broker from Orange County, California, who climbed the U.S. Bank Tower in Los Angeles in 2009. He's completed more than twenty climbs since then.

Leland was looking for "a new sport that didn't require a lot of time away from my kids. I didn't want to play golf. I used to play indoor soccer two or three times a week in competitive leagues until I was about forty. I don't play soccer anymore, and running is too hard on me. With stair climbing there are many more benefits to my physical and mental health than I could have ever imagined. I tore my quadricep muscle playing soccer several years ago and still have substantial scar tissue, but it hasn't inhibited me from climbing. I also want to live to be 107 years old so I can see the tri-centennial of the United States of America!"

Leland likes the fifty-five-story Figueroa at Wilshire Climb the best because "the steps are only 6.8 inches tall and I notice that my legs don't fatigue as quickly. The steps are also made of stamped steel, which I love, and that makes them bouncier. The stairwell is narrow enough for me to use both railings, which is what I prefer as opposed to only using the inside railing. I should also say that Scale the Strat in Las Vegas holds a special place in my heart. A dear friend of mine passed away two days before the Strat in 2013, so that climb will always have special significance to me as I honor and remember him each year. The AON Los Angeles is technically difficult, and it is challenging for me to establish any sort of rhythm climbing up that building. The steps are big and made of concrete, and the stairwell has only inside railings."

Leland trains by "going to the gym twice a week for strength and conditioning. I live in Orange County, so there aren't any tall buildings to practice in. There is a six-story parking garage in my hometown that I run up and down. When I can, I'll drive to Laguna Beach to train at Thousand Steps Beach (which is actually 219 steps according to my count). I'll train on the Jacob's Ladder, and when the Los Angeles stair climb events offer practice climbs downtown, I drive up there to train when I can."

As far as step-siblings go, Leland says, "I just love 'em all." He idolizes Ned Greene. Ned "is seventy years old and about my height (5'3"). He did the Willis Tower 103 floors in 17:40. He beat me in the San Diego twenty-floor sprint last year with a time of 2:18. He is showing me what can be done at age seventy."

Leland is big into music. While training and competing he listens to "100 percent EDM (electronic dance music). I find that most EDM tunes are around 120 bpm, so if you are stepping on beats two and four, you're right around 60 bpm, which is perfect for my long workouts on the Jacob's Ladder or jogging in my neighborhood. As a keyboardist, I like music that is mostly keyboard based: BT, Above & Beyond, Zedd, and Mat Zo.

"I'd just like to say that the beauty of stair climbing is that people of all shapes and sizes can excel at this sport. It's all about the power-to-weight ratio, and there are some petite girls (much smaller than me) who are blazing fast and can beat most of the guys. It's also a sport you can continue to do later in life, and as Ned Greene has shown, you can be very competitive in your seventies if that's what you want."

Harish Nambiar

Sweet Harish Nambiar is a forty-six-year-old engineer who completed his first climb, the ALA Fight for Air Climb in Oakbrook Terrace (a Chicago suburb), on February 13, 2011. He has completed nearly forty climbs to date, including several with his entire family.

He started climbing to motivate a family friend who was fighting lung cancer. "Growing up as a child, I was not gifted with any natural athletic talent. My activities were mostly confined to books, drawing and painting, and so forth. I envied the kids who were so good at athletics and sports. I did play with friends for fun and recreation, but that was the limit of my athletic activity.

"As an adult I exercised fairly regularly and was in decent shape physically. When our first child was born in December 2005, I spent time taking care of the baby and didn't have time to go to the gym. For about two years after that, I traveled a lot for work—four to six weeks at a time. All the restaurant food and no exercise added up quickly. In 2007 when I went to see my doctor for a physical, I had gained about forty pounds (I weighed 205, the most I've ever weighed). My cholesterol was high; my triglycerides were at 360. My doctor was ready to put me on a cholesterol medication. I told him to give me some time and promised to come back in six months.

"I took up running and registered for my first 5k. It was a great experience, and I was addicted. The same year I started running longer distances and competed in a half marathon. The next year, 2009, I ran the Chicago Marathon, my first. I loved the race experience. I've run in four Chicago Marathons so far, plus several half marathons, 5ks, and relay races.

"I went back to my doctor after a year of running. He was shocked to see the results. He could not believe it was really my report. I had lost forty pounds. My blood work was perfect. My good cholesterol had gone up to 45, my total cholesterol went down to 128, and my triglycerides went down to 80. I was ecstatic, and I promised myself that I would never let myself get back into that situation ever again.

"In 2010 October a dear family friend of ours who was sixty-seven years old was diagnosed with stage four lung cancer. Within a month of that, I got a postcard in the mail for the ALA Fight for Air Climb in Oakbrook. To this day I have no idea how they got my address or how I got the post card. I thought what a coincidence it was that our friend was fighting lung cancer, and I had this opportunity to help with lung disease. So I signed up, and that was the beginning of my climbing. Our friend passed away in May 2011. In 2012 I did the ALA circuit in his honor.

"During this time, I got to know the ALA staff all over the upper Midwest, including then-CEO of the Upper Midwest Harold Wimmer (the current national CEO of ALA). I came across several incredible world-class athletes and several amazing people who were brave and courageous in the face of adversities—people from all walks of life with one common cause: to lead a healthy and full life and make the earth a better place for generations to come. These people are so humble and caring; it has been such an eye opener. My life is richer with this sport."

Harish is a fan of the "power hour." He explains, "I am not fast. I like the endurance aspect. And Oakbrook is where it all started for me; it's a hometown event and will always have a special place for me." That said, he doesn't like the Milwaukee Power Hour. "It's forty-seven floors, so the break doesn't come soon enough between climbs, unlike a thirty-floor building. Also the stairs are steep, and the air is very dry and stale."

When asked about his stepfamily, Harish said "I have gotten to know hundreds of them through my association with this sport. I especially get to meet and spend more time with the ones in the Midwest. I am amazed at what great individuals they are and how much they genuinely care for each other."

His family inspires him first and foremost, followed by amazing people he's met from every walk of life, such as Mark Block. Harish says, "I am impressed that my sons, ages ten and seven, try to follow in my footsteps, and I'm honored to be their role model. My older son did two climbs in 2014, and he's doing the same two climbs this year as well. I am getting him involved in running as well. In 2015 at the Oakbrook ALA-FFAC, my whole family climbed for the first time. It was the first time for my wife and younger son. It was an unbelievable experience for us. This is hopefully just a start. I would love to see my children be active and strive to be the best they can be in anything they do."

Harish doesn't eat or drink anything before his races, since almost all of the runs and climbs happen by 7:00 a.m.

Harish's take on stair climbing? "This is one of the toughest sports. I am glad I stumbled onto it. This gives me something to do in the cold winter months in the Midwest. It has exposed me to incredible people. I consider my life to be richer with the introduction of this sport and the people involved in it."

Syd Arak

Seventy-year-old Syd is an attorney and adjunct law professor in Indianapolis. His first climb was the Bop to the Top Climb in Indianapolis in 1994. He's done it nineteen times since. Syd has climbed Willis twelve years in a row, and has had the good fortune to get into ESBRU seven times. He has completed more than seventy-five climbs.

"I was a runner and started doing the Bop to the Top as something different, without any special training. I enjoyed the challenge, realized I was good at it, and kept at it every year, but I didn't compete in any other climbs until 2004. My girlfriend climbed stairs at work for exercise, and we did some stair workouts together. Stair races were still pretty rare back then. I told her I wanted to do the Empire State Building Climb, but it was hard to get into. She suggested entering the Willis Climb since it was the tallest building in the country. Knowing how hard the thirty-six-floor Bop to the Top is, I thought she was crazy, but we did the Sears in 2004, and I've climbed it every year since."

Syd climbs for the same reason he still runs and bikes. "I'm still competitive and it's a way to force me to stay in shape and see where I'm at. For a long time I could track my improvement, but now that my times have started to slip, I'm starting to re-evaluate this, regardless of age group success. Also stair climbing does not lead to injury and is a great winter activity. Lastly, and not to be discounted, I've met so many terrific, supportive, and interesting people through this sport, and I've made lots of wonderful friends. By forming the West Coast Labels Team, Mark Trahanovsky created an atmosphere where there's always someone you know at every stair climb, which makes the events about the people as well as the climbs."

Syd's favorite climb is the Empire State Building RunUp—the way it used to be. "It was hard to get into, with a relatively small international field—about two hundred men and less than a hundred women. They had two mass starts for men and one for women into a narrow doorway, with narrow stairs, landings every floor that you had to run, and the finish outside with a sprint around the observation deck. It wasn't a charity event; it was run by the NY Road Runners. It was different and special, but isn't that way anymore. I was fortunate enough to be selected to compete for six years in a row, from 2006–2011."

Piero Dettin from Venice, Italy, inspires Syd. "He won my age group every year and was a legend. I could never beat him, but we became good friends and met for lunch every year before ESBRU and Sears in spite of the language barrier. When I finally did beat him, it was a great feeling of accomplishment."

Syd doesn't have a least favorite climb. "They are all painful. Some climbs are better run than others, and fortunately the charity climbs have become much more professional over the years. I've been fortunate enough to have some age-group success on a competitive level over the years, which I suppose has kept me hooked. I even was an overall winner in a local ALA triple climb a few years ago. But there's always somebody faster out there to keep me humble. I like to joke that my success is due to the difficulty my age-group competitors have getting up the stairs with their walkers and wheelchairs, but that isn't true at all. I'm heartened to see there are still plenty of competitive 'older' people who keep themselves in excellent shape out there. And, of course, there are still lots of younger folks to out-climb. Stair climbing is a great exercise for people of all ages; it's nonimpact and easy on your joints, at least on the way up. And it doesn't have to be competitive."

Mark Block

Fifty-year-old Mark Block tackled his first skyscraper in November 2010 via the SkyRise Chicago 2010 hand cycle competition. He has completed more than thirty climbs since.

Mark has quite a story. "I was in a car accident when I was twenty years old and paralyzed from my neck down. The doctors told my parents that if I survived, I would never move again, let alone walk. I was in the hospital for six months and eventually was able to walk again with the use of a leg brace and cane. Although still dependent upon the leg brace, I was able to complete fifteen miles of the Drake Relays Marathon by walking for eight hours and thirty-three minutes in 1988.

"My progress continued to a near-normal baseline, and I went on to return to work in sales, get married, and have children. I excelled in sales for many of the world's largest healthcare companies, but in June 2009 I fell and hit my head while loading boxes into my work vehicle. I sustained yet another SCI, my second, and a TBI [traumatic brain injury] too. I was sent to the Rehabilitation Institute of Chicago for complications of autonomic dysreflexia and left-sided paralysis, both of which I still struggle with. The lay term for my condition is ambulating quadriplegic: I have motor and sensory deficits in all four limbs, but I am able to walk.

"While I was being treated at RIC, I wanted to climb the Willis (Sears) Tower but was unable to climb stairs. My therapy team (MD/PT) allowed me to train for three weeks on the hand cycles under medical supervision. I completed the climb in the hand cycle division in thirty-six minutes by using my right arm only. I went back the following year and climbed the stairs during SkyRise 2011 and completed the climb in one hour and three minutes (in spite of the three broken ribs I incurred during a fall the previous day).

"I have since done the stairs of Willis three more times (as of February 2015) with assistance from my physical therapist from RIC who first helped me climb and train on stairs safely. The Willis Tower Climb is always my favorite because I was a patient at RIC, it raises funds for brain and spinal cord injury research at RIC, and I lead a team of disabled athletes, climbers, and hand cyclers on Team Altitude, including many former patients I met at RIC that are/were paralyzed like me. Also, Willis is the hardest and tallest of all the climbs, and it has the greatest meaning to me because of what RIC has helped me overcome."

Mark climbs because he remembers a time when he couldn't climb. "I climb for those who can't and to show myself and others that anything is possible when you try and when you have good people supporting you like the doctors, nurses, and therapists at RIC, and all my step-brothers and sisters from WCL who spot me at the climbs so I can push myself farther in a safe way."

Mark also rides recumbent trikes with a team called Adaptive Sports Iowa. "We train, race, and tour in the summer and ride in a group of thousands of riders across the state of Iowa in six days in an event called RAGRAI."

Mark has a special relationship with several step-siblings, including Karen Geninatti, John "Oz" Osborn, Scott Stanley, and Dave Schurtz. He is inspired by "former and current patients from RIC and other athletes from Adaptive Sports Iowa who I cycle with, and patients I have gotten to know from the On With Life brain injury center, where I was also treated. I think of my therapists and doctors who have supported me when others said I couldn't, and it inspires and motivates me. Each person who comes up to me before, during, or after a climb, many with tears in their eyes, and shares with me how my being there at a climb has touched them or motivated them totally inspires me to keep going!"

Mark doesn't listen to music when he works out. "Because of my injuries, balance disorder, and difficulty moving and concentrating, I need to focus. Focus is perhaps my biggest challenge—Karen Geninatti would agree. I don't use an iPod or any other device. My main focus is on picking up each individual foot and placing it on the step, as this is not automatic for me and takes a great deal of effort. When I get distracted I often trip and fall. Even people passing me or a loud noise can cause me to get distracted and fall. Karen counts the stairs out loud, and I try to stay focused on her voice."

I asked Mark to share his philosophy after all he's been through. "You never know what you can do until you try," he said. "If you listen to what other people tell you, you might not even try at all! If I had listened to what they were telling me when I was twenty years old, I would have given up and not be walking today. If I had listened to what others were telling me in 2009 after I got hurt again, I would have never gotten into stair climbing. I would never have met the many wonderful people who support me and help me climb to get better. Through climbing I have experienced being totally 'in the zone,' and I've had numerous peak performances that at one point in my life I thought I might never experience again. The sense of community and support I have received through climbing has not only helped me to get better physically—it has also helped me to look at life mentally in a more positive, optimistic way."

Margaret "Maggie" Lonergan

Twenty-seven-year-old Maggie Lonergan is a data scientist with an intense zeal for life. She is ranked the number forty-seven female climber in the world. She began her stair climbing ventures at the Hustle Up the Hancock Climb in 2012. She has competed in more than a dozen competitive climbs since.

"I started climbing while I was working in intelligence," she says. "Due to security requirements we didn't have Internet access in the building, and we weren't allowed to have cell phones. The weather was awful for a few months, which meant that going for a quick walk to break up the boredom was out of the question, so I took to hitting the stairs just to get out of the office."

Her favorite climb is the Willis Tower. "I have a deep personal connection with Sears. When I first learned about the climb, I was stuck in a rut, hating my job, knowing that I needed to do something different with my life but unsure of how to go about doing it. I found that the Sears Climb coincided with my sister's birthday (she lives in Chicago), and there were direct flights from O'Hare to Hong Kong, which made my plans to visit a friend in Hong Kong more realistic.

"Eventually those plans turned into taking an open-ended sabbatical, so the climb really marked the start of my year of wandering; I spent the next few months backpacking, and I eventually quit my intelligence job and took a few months to teach yoga, train for a marathon, and get my personal life together. The following November I was still a little unsettled, but I used the climb as a stopping-off point before I headed to San Francisco. I wanted to move there, but I had trouble justifying the move when I had no job, had blown through nearly all my savings, and had a very good job offer back in D.C. for a position I could realistically see myself loving.

"After the climb, I headed to San Francisco for a planned two-week vacation, found a job right away, and have been loving the California lifestyle ever since. Just before Sears the next year (2014, my third year in a row), I finally went back to D.C. It was my first trip back since I left for my two-week California vacation. I had to tie up some loose ends, say good-bye to some folks I feel reasonably sure I'll never see again, and apologize to friends who felt I had abandoned them when I never came home. While the 2014 climb was not my best, it felt like a good conclusion to my D.C. trip. This climb is brutal and really pushes you to dig deep; it was the first thing I did on my yearlong search for self, and it nicely book-ended it as I wrapped things up and fully transitioned into a much more settled life in San Francisco."

When I asked Maggie which climb she liked the least, she replied, "I haven't encountered a climb I wouldn't do again."

Maggie likes that stair climbing "forces you deep into your own body. One of the things that I love about competitive free diving is that you are forced to stay calm and present; otherwise you could drown. As long as you stay calm, you remain in control; any distraction could prove fatal. Climbing is the closest land-based activity I have found to this state of forced intense concentration. I can always find the same state while on my bike, but it requires a lot of effort to push myself to those limits and stay there. On the stairs you only need to focus on the stairs directly in front of you, your breathing, and your heartbeat. If you lose focus on any of those things, you blow up."

I loved that when I asked Maggie if there were any issues she needed to overcome to climb, her response was "laziness." (I can relate!) She said, "I train almost exclusively on the bike. Living in San Francisco I walk up hills a lot, which helps, but it's primarily cycling for my training. Sometimes I'll do breath-control work in the pool, which I think helps train my respiratory muscles, but it is primarily a good psychological training tool to simulate that feeling of not being able to catch your breath.

"My sister tags along on many of my physical adventures. She isn't in the greatest of shape, and I know these things (long bike rides, stair climbs, even half marathons) are really hard for her, but she always says yes when I ask if she wants to join me."

As for prerace rituals, Maggie loves "a sushi dinner the night before a race, or lox and toast for a prerace breakfast" but she remarks, "I don't freak out if I can't get either."

Maggie has some good advice for those who might be feeling stuck: "If you're stuck in a rut, you don't necessarily need a full plan to get yourself out of it. Every step you take is important; do things that are challenging to you, and eventually you'll have the confidence you need to make big decisions about your life. I remember thinking how dumb that sounded when I was really stuck, but by taking almost a year to focus entirely on doing things that scared and challenged me—including many physical challenges like stair climbing—I know that I am so much stronger than before. I now do things that I would have passed on years ago because I was too nervous to do them or unsure of how to proceed. I credit climbing for jump-starting that process, and I recommend it as an easy empowerment tool for anyone."

To be further inspired by Maggie, check out hiccupingyogi.com.

Sherri Breese

I first met Sherri Breese the night before my first Strat climb in 2014. She works in marketing, and her first climb was the Willis Tower in 2011. She has done well over a dozen climbs in her lifetime and is currently ranked number thirty-eight female climber in the world. "I started because my husband, Steve, was roommates with Brady Renshaw when we first started dating in 2010. They did the Willis Tower Climb with Brady's girlfriend and powerhouse, Kristin Frey. I was jealous that they got to go downtown and hang out at the top of the Willis Tower. The next year I signed up so I wouldn't be left out! I like the races, climbing with my husband, and seeing my step-siblings. I also like traveling to downtown Chicago, and I have been to Seattle, Vegas, and New York."

She likes AON Chicago best "because it is ten steps, left turns the whole way, so it's easy to find a rhythm. I like Willis because longer events play to my strength since I am a marathon runner." The 300 N. LaSalle Building, Chicago, is her least favorite. "I like the relaxed atmosphere, but I don't like the shallow, carpeted stairs, and long landings."

Sherri is inspired by her husband, Steve, who "always has a positive attitude and pushes me to be my best. I'm grateful to Brady and Kristin for showing me proper stair-climbing techniques. And a big thanks to David Hanley, Mark, and PJ for all the stats and admin work they do. Madeline Ronk and Mark Block have overcome amazing obstacles to get to where they are today, because they refuse to give up."

I asked Sherri about how she prepares for a climb. "I used to eat pasta the night before a climb like I do for a running race, but found this to be too heavy for a climb," she told me. "I now eat a salad the night before a race. The morning of a race, I wake up four hours before the race to eat breakfast, which consists of half a banana plus a granola bar, toast, or crackers. I then go back to bed. I like to have four hours for my food to digest before a climb."

If thirty-three-year-old Sherri had a number on her racing jersey, she says, "It would be two because I am currently climbing for two! Baby Breese has been to the top of the Empire State Building and the Hancock Building in Chicago."

What does Sherri want to share with those who have never tried stair climbing? "Stair climbing is a very challenging sport because you need both power and endurance. It is lower-impact than running but a great lower and upper body workout, which makes it great cross-training for other sports. Plus, the races are fun, and I have met a great group of people!"

Alex Workman

"Super competitive" in his own words, soon-to-be forty-year-old Alex Workman is a stair-climbing machine. His nicknames are "The Schenectady Express" or "Calf Man."

An engineer by trade, Alex is president of the U.S. Stair Climbing Association. His first climb was the Albany Corning Tower in 2011. He has done four dozen lifetime climbs and is currently ranked fourteenth in the world among male climbers.

"A coworker climbed the Corning Tower in 2006 and came in second. It piqued my interest since it seemed like it would be something I'd be good at. But it wasn't until 2011 that I found the time and courage to try it. My goal was to beat my coworker's time from 2006. At the end of the race, I came in fourth overall with a time of 5:23, which was just a few seconds slower than my coworker at 5:18, but still really competitive. However, I was totally blown away by the first and second place climbers; the winner, David Tromp, was nearly a minute ahead of me with 4:30, and second place Tim Van Orden wasn't too far behind with 4:38. Afterward, I looked them up online and found out they were two of the top climbers in the U.S. I also realized that I had gone to college with David at Clarkson University. I knew he looked familiar, but he was seventy pounds lighter—no joke! At that moment my stair-climbing quest began."

Alex's favorite climb is City Place in Hartford, Connecticut. "It is a short race, just over three minutes, which plays to my strengths. Plus the stairwell is perfectly configured, eleven step flights and double rails, which makes this a *fast* race." His least favorite climb is the Empire State Building RunUp: "It's the most difficult climb for me. It has a mass start, which screws up my rhythm, has lots of flats with running and I'm not a runner, and is the second tallest climb in the United States and I'm a sprinter. Basically this race plays to all of my weaknesses."

Alex has nerve damage in his foot, which prevents him from running long distances. "Fortunately climbing stairs doesn't aggravate it," he says. "I also have a pretty severe case of asthma. If I didn't take lung medication, I couldn't climb competitively."

He trains by doing "lots of lunges and stairwell sprints." He adds, "I also spend a lot of time on my Precor stepper machine (Precor C776I). For cross training I prefer rowing and cycling, which both mimic certain aspects of stair climbing. On my rest days I like using the elliptical machine. I have a newfound respect for rowers." For a prerace ritual, Alex does burpees. "They are great way to warm-up," he says.

As for Alex's step-siblings, he says, "Two Davids come to mind. The first David is David Tromp, who I've already mentioned. We have a lot in common besides stair climbing. Believe it or not, when we run into each other, we rarely even talk about racing! The second David is David Hanley. He has great sense of humor and is passionate about stair climbing. We get along quite well. Last but not least, I have to give a shout out to my Tower Masters teammates; we're the East Coast's preeminent stair-climbing squad."

Sproule Love, ranked number ten in the world, also inspires Alex. "He is a climbing legend."

Alex's take on stair climbing? "If a heavyset thirty-eight-year-old asthmatic with bum feet can climb stairs competitively, so can you. I was just average at endurance sports when I started climbing competitively at age thirty-five. My mantra is 'A steady pace wins the race.' "

Visit Alex and the U.S. Stair Climbing Association at www.tower runningusa.com.

Nelson Quong

One of the kindest souls in competitive climbing belongs to Nelson Quong. Forty-nine-year-old Nelson is a fatal accidents analyst for the California Highway Patrol who did his first climb in Sacramento in November 2009. He's done about two-dozen climbs since.

Nelson saw a short blurb about the Empire State Building RunUp years ago in *Runner's World*. "I promised myself if we ever had a climb in Sacramento, I would do it, never expecting we would have one! I also thought it would be great cross-training for my bike racing. I ended up loving it so much that I used my cycling to train for stair racing instead."

Nelson was an amateur bike racer for seventeen years, but that ended when he sustained a serious knee injury. He shared with me what happened: "I had an appointment with my optometrist the morning of November 12, 2010. I took my climbing clothes, headphones, and gloves along, intending to hit the college stairs afterward. Because my optometrist dilated my eyes, he strongly suggested I go home and rest my eyes first, or I could risk falling and hurting myself on the stairs. Once home I decided to lie down for an hour before climbing. I was just falling asleep when a coworker called to ask a work question. Startled and with my vision blurry, I jumped out of bed and ran at a full sprint to answer the phone. I hit the doorway hard with my knee and finished the call before I noticed my knee was really wet (I didn't realize it was blood right away). I bandaged it and went to climb the college stairs. The pain in my leg increased over the next two days, and by the third day, I couldn't bend it. I finally went to see a doctor. It was misdiagnosed for six months before an MRI revealed severe tendon and cartilage damage."

Nelson says that before his knee injury, his main form of training was cycling, and he also trained with weights at the gym and climbed at a local college parking structure. "Since I was injured, though, I haven't been able to cycle, but I still do restricted workouts in the gym and climb the parking structure when my pain level is down. The structure is only five floors, but it is the tallest staircase I have access to, so it has special meaning to me.

"My favorite climb is still the Sacramento Climb because it was my first stair race, and I was surprised how well I did despite how horrible I felt. A close second favorite would be AON because that's where I first nervously approached Mark to wish him luck and tell him I had seen him in climbing videos. That is also the first race I did with you, Jane! Originally I had pretty severe social anxiety. Bike racing was a pretty insular activity. I did meet some good friends through it, but there really wasn't the same camaraderie or closeness there is in stair climbing. Stair climbing has helped me live outside the box. I've had pretty severe social anxiety most of my life—I used to have a very hard time leaving my house and even used to go running at night so no one would see me. I never would have imagined I'd be flying all over the country and have great friends from all over the world. Stair climbing opened up the world for me.

"At first, I climbed to cross-train for cycling and because I loved the extreme mental and physical challenge of it. That's still true, but now I also climb for the wonderful bonds I've formed with my teammates. They are truly bonds formed by mutual suffering!"

When asked who inspires him, Nelson said, "That's a great question—and a tough one. You know that you inspire me! Also many of our step-sibs inspire me for so many different reasons. We've all had such different challenges to overcome. I honestly believe that's one of the reasons we're drawn to the sport and to each other. In stair climbing, everyone suffers, but we are the ones that always get up and fight."

Nelson doesn't have a particular prerace ritual. "I try not to adopt any superstitions or rituals because I travel for most of my races, so I don't want to adopt anything I can't easily replicate in another city. I don't want it to throw off my race. That being said, I do tend to look up to the sky at the moon the night before a race. I was very close to my grandmother. When I was little, she would babysit me, and we would sit on a step and look at the moon together before bedtime. She's been gone for many years, but this still comforts me to this day."

If we had numbers on our jerseys, Nelson says he would choose eight or thirteen. "Eight is good luck in Chinese, and thirteen represents overcoming challenges or 'bad luck' while racing." He likes to listen to hard rock while working out.

"Climbing means even more to me now than it did before my injury," Nelson says. "Although I'm climbing much slower now, I actually think

I'm pushing myself mentally more than when I was healthy. Before, I knew that if I slowed down, the pain would eventually go away. Now, even if I slow down, I know the pain will only drop back to the same level it's at every day when I'm not climbing. I use this knowledge to keep pushing myself. In stair climbing, we all suffer and push ourselves despite our circumstances. To me, that's both the challenge and the beauty of the sport!"

Sarah Johnson

Sarah Johnson is an accounting supervisor for an oil and gas company. The forty-six-year-old did her first climb on March 24, 2012, at the ALA Race, First City Tower, Houston, Texas, and has done more than fifteen climbs since. "I started climbing stairs at work to lose weight and get in better shape. I did that for about three years, and then I remembered a *60 Minutes* episode I saw as a kid about the Empire State Building Climb. I wondered if this event still happened, and I soon discovered the worldwide sport of stair climbing."

Sarah says she continues to climb because "it's the best cardio conditioning there is." She told me, "When I started climbing, my knees hurt from an old running injury. The more I climbed, the stronger my knees got. I now have no knee issues at all. I am currently working through a hip injury, though."

Unlike most of her step-siblings, the Willis Tower is her favorite climb. "I have only climbed it once, but I loved climbing such an iconic building, and I felt particularly good the day of that climb. The party and view at the top was also a great payoff."

Sarah says, "I am very passionate about my overall conditioning and strength. I love my boot camp and I also love trail running. I train with my boot camp regularly, and I climb in the twenty-five-floor building where I work. I also do yoga, spinning, and trail running."

Sarah met Scott Stanley and Dan Dill at her first race. "They are my Team Texas brothers, and they inspire me with their passion for life and fitness. I am inspired by older athletes, in particular women athletes, who live life with passion and are forever discovering the depth of their strength."

Before a race, Sarah likes to "wake up super early, have my breakfast and coffee, warm up with a prerace workout, and flood my mind with positive thoughts. Then I just relax and have fun."

For anyone interested in stair climbing, Sarah says, "Stair climbing is something you can do and reap huge gains regardless of your skill level."

Stephen Marsalese

I had seen fifty-year-old Stephen Marsalese at climbs, but I didn't really get to know this gentle man until after the World Trade Center Climb in 2015. He is a doorman in New York City and did his first climb at the Empire State Building in 1996. He has completed seventy-five climbs in his career. He had been a runner, and he wanted to do something different for a change. "I did the Empire State Building RunUp in 1996, and I was hooked! It's an amazing workout, and I love to race."

When it comes to a favorite climb, for Stephen it's a tie between the Bennington Monument and the Empire State Building. He is not fond of the Corning Tower in Albany, New York.

He trains on the StairMaster at the gym twice a week. "I also do spinning at the gym three to four times a week. When the weather is nice, I do outdoor stairs on my way to work—120 stairs, about eight flights. I do that seven times, all out, about twice a week. I'm not running much now; I only run in the spring and summer, two to three times a week, up to twenty-five miles a week."

Stephen's favorite step-sibling is Michael Karlin, who he says is "great to chat with!" He is also inspired by "my family and Bruce Springsteen." He drinks "a nice strong cup of coffee" before races. The coffee must work—he's currently the number thirty-six male climber in the world.

"I love to race. To put on a number and race up the stairs, fight through the pain, and pull yourself on the railings is an amazing feeling, and every race is different. Then when you get to the top and look down below to see what you climbed . . . well, everyone in the world should experience that at least once in his or her lifetime!"

Michael Carcieri

Sixty-four-year-old Michael Carcieri's given name is John, but he says, "My father was the only person, other than the nuns at school, who called me John. To everyone else I was always Michael (or 'Hey you!')." Michael, an accountant, is currently controller at Hilton Universal City, California. His first climb was the U.S. Bank Tower in 2008. When asked how many climbs he's completed, Michael says, "I've lost count, but nowhere near enough."

He started climbing in 2007 when a vice president from Union Bank came to his office in Pasadena to take him to lunch. "My office was at the top of a fourth-floor walk-up with no elevators. I two-stepped the whole way. She asked if I had ever heard of the U.S. Bank/YMCA stair climb, and I replied no. I later Googled it and was going to do it that year, but then decided that I had a lot of good excuses not to, so I passed on it. I thought about it all year, though, and decided I had to man-up the next year in 2008."

His favorite climb? The CFF Climb in November. "There's not many in my age group, so I might have a better chance at a medal. I'm vain, okay?" His least favorite is the Willis Tower. "Absolute torture! I will have to conquer it, however, before I finally quit stair racing."

Michael is motivated to climb because of his father. "My father was quite ill with advanced type 2 diabetes in 1990 and had to have a leg amputated. My dad was devastated. This was a man who walked to work when I was young back in the 1950s and early 60s. He was so strong— he drove a forklift and lifted heavy freight all day. Now he was 'out of the game.' In 1991 he was advised to have his second leg amputated, and he decided he didn't want to go out one limb at a time. He told me he had had enough. He went off dialysis and was dead in ten days. He was sixty-one.

"I thought about the gift of mobility and how my dad felt so lost without his ability to move around. I think of him every time I run the stairs. I also think of my mother who died six years ago on Mother's Day, disabled by a stroke. She was another one who could walk over five miles to work without a peep. My role models are my parents, the people who gave me the ability to walk and run. Climbing is difficult; a simple walk around the park might suffice for some, but not for me. I feel more alive when I am pushing the grim reaper further into the rearview mirror."

Michael used to love scuba diving, and he became an assistant to an instructor for the Barnacle Busters scuba club. But then his asthma got the better of him, and he could no longer take the chest pressure. Next he started Masters Swimming.

"I was never fast," he says, "but I enjoyed exhausting myself at every workout. I never thought I would swim two to three miles per training session three times a week. And now my newest poison is trail running. I'm currently training for the Verdugo 10k in May, blame it on Jeff Dinkin. I had to run out of excuses for being too old, too sore, saying my hips hurt, my asthma blocks my airways, or my heart does not pump well enough. I do have a heart murmur—I can't hear it, but the doctor can. My heart still has a bad valve, but it works well enough to keep me going up two steps at a time."

As for training, Michael says, "I prefer to train with the group. I need to try to keep up with the gazelles, even if only for a few floors. The challenge of practicing with stronger runners helps me improve."

When asked about his step-siblings, Michael's reply was: "Well, I feel a connection with you; you're a no-nonsense, you-are-who-you-are kind of person. You could walk around the park, but you push it at stair races instead. I also admire and very much appreciate the helpful pointers from Lisa, Stan, Veronica, and Jeff Dinkin. Jeff has given me so many constructive pointers, from my great pair of New Balance Minimus (most comfortable racing shoes ever) to suggesting that I consider trail running since he and I usually meet up every year at the Tram Road Race in Palm Springs. I have met so many kind people who are always supportive and happy to see me and other 'non-rockets' who show up for the practices. Feeling included is important. I feel a bit guilty if I don't remember all the names, but I remember the kind faces—between the rivers of sweat, that is."

He is also inspired by James Masoner. "I always look for him at practices and the races; he's a guy who could hang it up but doesn't. Johnny Ravello is also a very gifted guy who needs to stay with it—he has a talent not to be wasted."

Michael always puts a wad of Dentyne cinnamon gum on each side of his upper gum, which he says keeps his mouth from drying out during the races. When I questioned him about his musical choices, he said, "I don't use an iPod. I just have a very varied play list in my head—it could be AC/DC or some similar headbanger, fast-beat rock. I leave the country music for mellow times."

Michael shared these thoughts of encouragement. "Do not ever sell yourself short—you have more in the tank if you're willing to dig deep for it. There is no magic to this; the best runners have strong minds to drive their bodies. Always seek out stronger runners and work to keep up with them, even if only for a short burst. You will improve. I would never have imagined feeling as alive as I do after races such as U.S. Bank in September."

Hal Carlson

Hal is a retired fire chief from Aurora, Illinois. At the age of sixty-three, he is currently the sixty-seventh fastest climber in the world and has completed over ninety climbs. His first climb was the Hustle Up the Hancock in Chicago on February 23, 2003.

He started climbing when he was recovering from a running injury. "We had a fire in our local high-rise (twenty stories), and I was surprised at how hard it was to run up the stairwell." Hal says he climbs because "it's an excellent work out, it's great cross training for runners, and it's nice to compete in shorts and a T-shirt in the winter." He trains by doing stairs as often as possible, using the StairMaster, running, rowing, and biking.

Hal's favorite climb is the Empire State Building. "I love the stair layout, the international field, the history and tradition—and of course, it's in New York."

Hal says, "The stair climbing community is a tight group. I have made many good friends along the way. When I first started climbing, there was a man named John who had lost hundreds of pounds—he had a website called WayTooFat.com." Hal is also inspired by elites such as Henry Wigglesworth, Dan Ackerman, Syd Arak, and Ned Greene.

No stranger to overcoming challenging obstacles, Hal told me, "I broke my neck on July 4, 2005, competing in a race in Alaska called Mt. Marathon. This put me in a neck collar for almost six months, but I was still able to compete in the Willis and Milwaukee stair climbs in November."

Ned Greene

Seventy-one-year-old Ned Greene still works as a dentist in Lincoln, Nebraska.

His first climb was the Trek Up the Tower in Omaha in 2009. He's done about two dozen climbs so far. "I started stair climbing in earnest when I had to stop running because of extensive back problems. I used to run one marathon per year, and I ran the Boston Marathon several times. Stair climbing does not bother my poor back."

Ned continues to climb because he says the one thing everyone needs is a purpose! "Stair climbing gives me a purpose—a purpose to train hard, and a purpose to be good at something. I want to be good at something that is athletic and health-related.

"Willis Tower is my favorite climb because it is long," Ned says. "Older people do better at endurance events rather than shorter sprint-type events." That said, Ned isn't crazy about the Stratosphere. "I didn't know how to pace myself very well, and I didn't like waiting in that wind tunnel for thirty minutes."

Ned loves road biking. "Especially biking uphill. Biking and stair climbing go very well together. My most important event every year is the Mt. Evans Hill Climb in Colorado. Stair climbing makes me a better uphill biker, which in turn makes me a better stair climber. Another purpose! Like stairs, biking (cycling) is great for lower back problems."

Running real stairs—sixteen flights two to three times a week—is how Ned trains, plus using the StairMaster stair stepper at his health club two or three times a week. He finds it harder on the weekends due to time constraints. "Starting about now, I am slowly transitioning to more biking, and I'll start training for the Willis Tower in early September."

Ned, the top climber in the United States in the 70–79 AG, likes to listen to Eminem while he climbs.

Martin Pedersen

Thirty-eight-year-old Martin Pederson from Denmark is a technical assistant who did his first climb in 2011 and has completed more than two-dozen climbs since. He's ranked the fortieth best climber in the world right now.

"It was a complete coincidence that I got started with stair climbing. I was looking at information about New York City in December 2010, as I was planning on going there for a holiday in the summer of 2011. I searched for info on the Empire State Building, and the third or fourth result was a link to the Empire State Building RunUp. I had had the chance to walk up the stairs from the eighth floor to the eighty-sixth floor on a previous visit to the ESB and had started running a few months earlier, so I decided to click on the link just to see what it was about. The website stated that applications for registering for the race were open only for the week, and there were one or two days left to apply.

"At that time you had to write a short essay as part of your application, so I wrote a short story about who I was, what my fitness level was, and why I wanted to do the race. Upon completing the application, I was informed that I would get an answer by the first full week of January (the race was on February 1st). I pretty much forgot about sending the application and didn't give it much thought when I hadn't received an answer at the end of the first full week of January. But then, during the middle of the following week, I received an email from the organizers saying that I had been accepted. Wow! I didn't have a valid passport, hadn't made any travel arrangements, and didn't have any stair-climbing experience. A few hectic weeks later and with a brand new passport, I set out for New York. And the rest is history, as they say."

Martin told me that his first climb was a result of his wish to travel. He went on to say, "When I found out that other stair climbs were held all over the world, it was a great way to combine my travels and my new desire to be fit—and stay fit. I know myself well enough to know that I need some sort of goal to keep myself motivated, and stair climbs are a perfect way to help me stay motivated. Getting to know quite a few people in the United States and be able to spend time with them has helped me to stay motivated to be healthy and fit enough to do stair climbs."

Martin says the Willis Tower Climb in Chicago is "brutal and steep." He's only done it once and told me, "Maybe I just had a bad day, but really steep steps are not my favorite thing. I'm too short."

Martin doesn't haven't access to any stairwells in the area where he lives. "For the most part I run, bike, or use a cross-trainer. Basically I do a lot of cardio workouts. Sometimes I wear a backpack with twenty pounds of extra weight when I bike around a short loop in my city that has some incline. In the weeks before a race, if I have the chance, I travel two miles by train to Copenhagen to train in a building with sixteen floors."

Martin says that different kinds of climbers inspire him. "Some of the climbers have incredible stories of weight loss, while others have issues with injuries, pain, heart attacks, cancer, and so forth, which they need to overcome to be able to climb. I have struggled with my weight, so I can relate to some of the issues. In cases where serious illnesses are involved, I can only be amazed of the willpower of some people; I find this to be highly inspirational, along with the super elites of stair climbing. Every stair climber knows the feeling of exhaustion after a climb. Some of the elites are on a fitness level that just boggles my mind. They inspire me to keep pushing myself when I work out and not become disillusioned about my own ability."

According to Martin, the stair-climbing communities in Europe and the United States are two very different things at this point. "The European scene is made up of a larger share of what you would call elite athletes, meaning athletes coming from other sports such as track and field, cross country, running, cycling, and mountain running—sports they are already highly skilled in. If you want to be in the top of any European races, you have to be really, really good. Most races are organized as 'races,' not primarily as a fund-raisers as most races are in the U.S."

Steve Coyne

I had met Chicago police officer Steve Coyne at other climbs, but I didn't get to know him until after we did the One World Trade Center Climb in 2015. Steve asked me what he had to do to get a team West Coast Labels jersey. I asked him what his time was and it was better than mine, so I told him I'd recommend him getting one to Mark.

Steve has completed more than thirty climbs since his first climb, the Sears Tower, in 2012.

"When I started, I climbed just to climb, just to see if I could make it. My time was a nonissue. Since the Triple Dawg Dare Climb in Oklahoma City in 2014, I've really 'stepped up' my training. That's where I met a few climbers from our Training Buds Facebook page in Chicago.

"A friend from grammar school asked me to join her team for the AON Building Climb in 2012. I had never done a climb before. My then-seven-year-old wanted to climb with daddy, so he and I did the Hustle Up the Hancock Half Climb, the U.S. Bank in Los Angeles, and now I climb for fitness. I've lost about fifty pounds since December 2013. I have a degenerative disc, and sometimes I really have to work past the pain and stretch out for over an hour before a workout or a climb. It's relatively minor compared to what I've seen others overcome.

"Stair climbing, especially when I work out at Swallow Cliff, is almost therapeutic. I go there, put my music on, and climb. It helps me forget about the daily stresses of life. I've worked hard at stair climbing, and I've seen a lot of improvements. I cut my time at U.S. Bank from 30:52 in to 2012 to 17:30 in 2015."

Steve says the Dallas 9/11 Memorial Climb is one of his favorites. "It's only open to police and firefighters, and we climb in full uniform/gear. Everything is based on the times of the WTC on 9/11. It's 110 flights of stairs (fifty-five floors twice). It's an untimed event. I play my bag-pipes with Dallas area police/fire Pipes and Drums during the opening ceremony."

In 2014, Steve met step-sister Sue Glaser at a climb in Oklahoma. "She introduced me to a lot of people at the climbs and on Facebook. She's been encouraging and supportive—she's like that with everyone. Since Okla-homa City, I've met Sue in Las Vegas, Dallas, New York, Chicago, and Greenville, South Carolina. My wife and I took her out for Chicago-style pizza after the Presidential Towers Climb this year."

Steve is inspired by many of his stepfamily. "Especially the climbers who are older than I am," he says. "It's great to see climbers in their mid-forties through sixties not only climbing, but excelling in the sport. Ninety-nine per-cent of athletes in their twenties and thirties couldn't get times like some of them. Also Mark Block and Cowboy George Burnham—it's amazing what Mark has overcome to continue climbing and to see George in his seventies do more climbs than anyone else."

Steve races with his iPod blaring heavy metal, when permitted. He puts a dab of Vapor Rub under each nostril to help him breathe better.

"I've met a lot of great people from all over, I've gotten to travel to a few places I normally wouldn't have, I've raised money for great causes, and I'm now in the best shape of my life. I'm in even better shape than in high school, college, or when I was boxing."

He says it was truly an honor to get a WCL shirt from Mark, and he's worn it for his last several climbs.

David Garcia

David Garcia is a thirty-seven-year-old television producer and prolific blogger in Los Angeles. "My first race was the ALA Fight for Air Climb in LA in 2012. In 2010 I started what would become a lifelong journey to lose weight and get healthy. At the time, I weighed over four hundred pounds. In about a year's time, I lost 160 pounds through diet and exercise, which I've kept off ever since. One of my weight loss habits was to try new things—whether foods, workouts, or mindsets.

"In 2011 I began eyeballing the StairMaster at my gym. It intimidated me, but I pushed myself to start using it. I started with just five minutes and slowly increased the time. I began noting, after each climb, how many floors I had climbed, and then I would go home and look up a skyscraper somewhere in the country that was the same height. Seeing photos of these tall buildings and knowing I climbed the equivalent inspired me to keep going, and soon I began challenging myself to climb on the StairMaster the equivalent of landmark buildings around the world. In a few months I had climbed the equivalent of the Burj Khalifa, Willis Tower, Chrysler Building, and Petronas Towers—the list goes on and on. I don't remember where I first heard about an actual stair-climb race, but the idea stuck in my head. If I was climbing buildings hypothetically at the gym, why couldn't I do it in real life, too? So I signed up for that first AON Center Climb, and I worked my ass off to prepare. I was terrified on the big day, looking up at that looming sixty-three-story building, but the feeling of pride and accomplishment I got on the roof afterward was overwhelming. It brought me to tears. I had done something that, just a few years prior, at four hundred pounds, would've been nearly impossible. It makes my heart race just thinking about it!"

David's favorite climb is the AON Center because "that's where I popped my stair-racing cherry." Otherwise, he says he loves traveling and conquering new buildings much more than doing the same ones again.

When I asked David why he climbs, he gave me several strong reasons. "I climb because the races require so much focus and dedication, and I like having events to work toward. Stair racing keeps me on track with my health and fitness goals, and it's a huge reason why I've been able to maintain my 160-pound loss. I climb because it's so challenging, so grueling, so intense, and therefore so rewarding. I climb because I like getting access to skyscraper rooftops and penthouse office suites—where the finish lines are—and access to those places is nearly impossible outside of a race setting. I climb because I've met an astounding, inspiring network of friends—many of whom are in this book—and I've never felt so welcomed and embraced in a team-like setting. Mostly, though, I race because I like proving to myself, again and again, that I am capable of extraordinary things, and I am worth the hard work and sacrifice needed to compete in such a strenuous sport."

David went on to say, "I'm not the fastest climber, and I probably never will be, and I'm fine with that. Now that I've lost and kept off the weight, my largest issues are mental ones. Starting up the stairs at the beginning of the race requires a lot of physical strength and endurance, but I also focus just as much on my attitude. This means encouraging myself, squashing thoughts of doubt or sabotage, and staying positive from the first floor to the last."

David told me he doesn't train too much on actual stairs because he doesn't like the repetition. "Once a week I'll train in a stairwell, or on some of the public stairways in the hilly parts of LA. I'll work out five other times during any given week, and some of that is cardio and weightlifting that targets the leg muscles that are engaged in climbing. But generally I switch it up—running, lifting, aerobic classes, swimming. I try to never do the same thing two days in a row."

David, like Kathleen Schwarz, has "worn the same pair of underwear at every race for the past year." He is "constantly tweaking" his workout playlist, but some of his favorites include "What I've Done" (Linkin Park), "Geronimo" (Sheppard), "It's Not Over Yet" (For King & Country), and "Army of Me" (Bjork).

"Had you told me five years ago that I would become so heavily invested in such an extreme sport in my mid-thirties, I would have laughed at you. I've never excelled at physical activity historically, and I never thought I ever would. But I kept an open mind and ended up falling into something I love. I want to encourage your readers to keep an open mind, too. They'll never know where a new experience might lead. Don't be afraid to try new things. The first time I stepped on a StairMaster, over four years ago, I certainly didn't think I'd become a nationally-ranked stair racer with twenty races under my belt, but that's what happened—because I was open-minded."

David writes about his struggles and successes at www.keepitupdavid .com and @keepitupdavid on Twitter and Instagram.

CPSIA information can be obtained
at www.ICGtesting.com
Printed in the USA
FSOW02n0811190516
20536FS